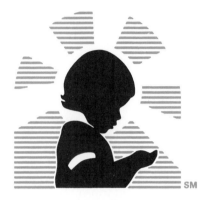

^{SM}

St. Jude Children's Research Hospital

ALSAC • Danny Thomas, Founder

FROM HIS PROMISE

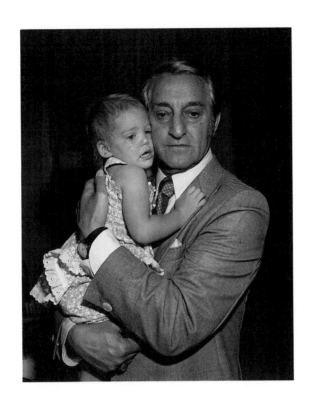

FROM
HIS
PROMISE

A History of ALSAC and
St. Jude Children's Research Hospital

GUILD BINDERY PRESS
MEMPHIS

Published in Memphis, Tennessee
by Guild Bindery Press, Inc.

Library of Congress Cataloging in Publication Data

From His Promise: A History of ALSAC and St. Jude
Children's Research Hospital/Author—1st ed. in the U.S.A.
        p.   cm.
        I. Title
        ISBN 1-55793-051-1
                CIP

Editor and Publisher: Randall Bedwell
Written and compiled by: Palmer Thomason Jones
Executive Editor: David Yawn
Contributing Editors: Robbin Brent, Trent Booker, Robert
Holmes, Trey Horst, Mel Goldsmith
Photo Researcher and Captions: Paul Parham
Researcher: Catherine Cline

ALSAC Liaison: Paul Parham

Jacket Design: Pat Patterson and Greg Hastings,
Patterson Graham Design
Page Layout and Design: Beverly Cruthirds,
Cruthirds Design

published in the United States by

GUILD BINDERY PRESS
Post Office Box 38099
Memphis, Tennessee 38183
email: guildmedia@aol.com

First Edition

10   9   8   7   6   5   4   3   2   1

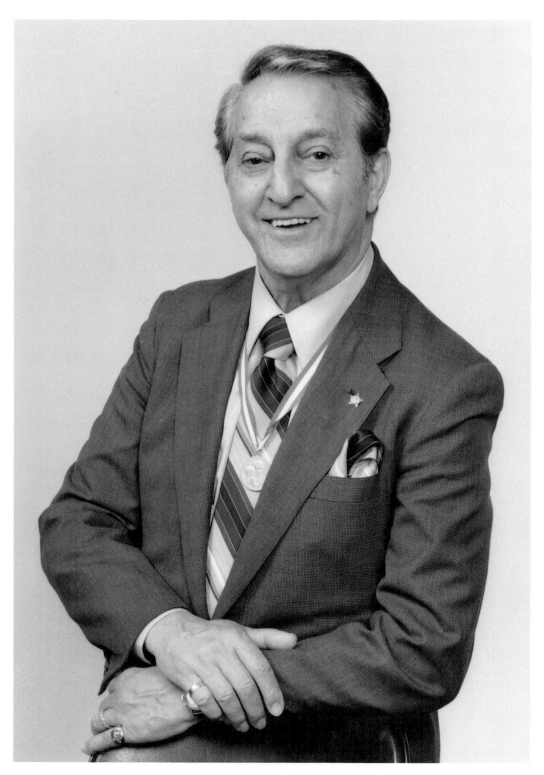

In Memory of Danny Thomas
1912 — 1991
Entertainer and Humanitarian

ACKNOWLEDGMENTS

Editorial oversight and review of the manuscript were provided by Albert Joseph and Judy Habib. Their experience both as respected professionals in the world of publishing and as members of the Board of Directors and Governors of ALSAC-St. Jude Children's Research Hospital was invaluable in the preparation of the manuscript.

Paul Parham, ALSAC's former director of communications, deserves special credit. He conceived this project and shepherded it through all stages. His additional research and interviews, preparation of four revisions, selection of photographs, writing of captions and many hours of time devoted to this book were given without compensation as a labor of love. Most of the research for this book came from the Paul Parham Archive Room which was dedicated to him after his retirement in 1995 after 19 years of service.

Additional thanks for their keen proofing and insightful comments go to Sheila Bonaiuto, Jerry Chipman, George Shadroui, Ruth Ann Skaff and Elizabeth Todd of the ALSAC-St. Jude staff.

Unless otherwise credited, all photographs are from the Biomedical Communications Department of St. Jude Children s Research Hospital and the ALSAC archives. Jerry Luther, John Zacher and Jere Parobek, and Constance Coleman were a tremendous help in sorting through the more than 15,000 photographs reviewed for this book.

Kathy Connelly and the Communications Department of ALSAC provided administrative assistance and greatly facilitated the preparation and transmittal of the manuscript during the review process.

Thanks also go to those who granted interviews on the earlier years of the organization, particularly to Albert Joseph, Baddia J. Rashid, LaVonne Rashid and Janet Roth.

In preparation of the text, extensive use was made of material from ALSAC's earlier history, *A Dream Come True*, ©1983, and in the ALSAC archives.

As with all attempts at recording history, *From His Promise* could not include the names of all the loyal, dedicated volunteers, staff, patients and parents who have contributed to this story. Those whose stories have been selected and named are meant to represent all whose experience at St. Jude Children's Research Hospital and ALSAC have run a gamut from despair to elation, from despondency to hope and from the early concerns about death and dying to today's emphasis on life and living. *From His Promise* owes them all a debt of gratitude.

Contents

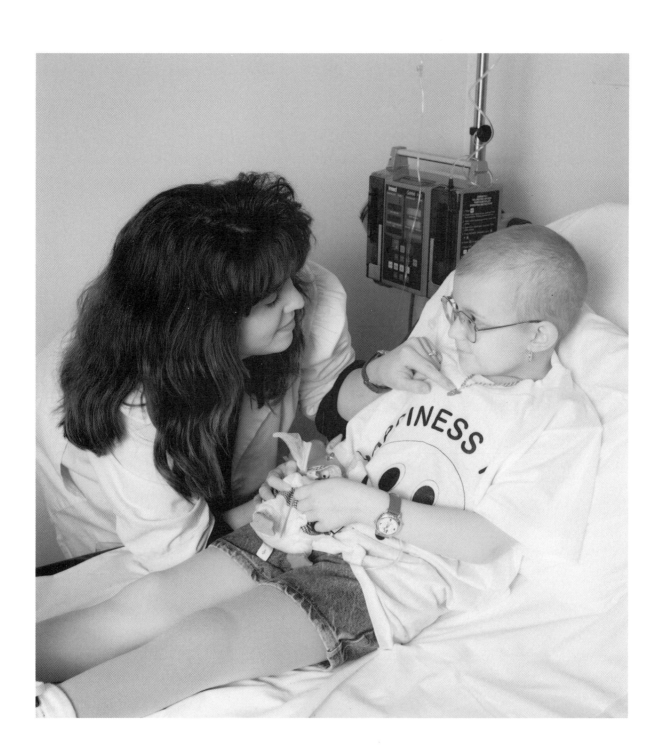

A Promise Made

"Help me find my place in life and I will build you a shrine where the poor and the helpless and the hopeless may come for comfort and aid."

These words, uttered in a Detroit church by a young Danny Thomas as a plea to St. Jude for guidance, have changed the way the world looks at childhood cancer. It was on this promise that St. Jude Children s Research Hospital was built the first institution established for the sole purpose of conducting basic and clinical research into catastrophic childhood diseases, mainly cancer. Since its opening in 1962, St. Jude has admitted more than 14,000 children from 47 states and 55 foreign countries. Its reputation, however, is founded on the success of its revolutionary treatment methods. In a little more than three decades, St. Jude physicians and scientists have succeeded in rewriting the medical textbooks that categorized childhood cancer, particularly leukemia, as incurable.

When St. Jude opened its doors in Memphis, Tennessee, in the early 1960s, a diagnosis of childhood cancer was a virtual death sentence. In 1962, approximately 95 out of 100 children stricken with cancer died. Despite their best efforts, the medical community could offer little more than pain relief for children with cancer. Doctors, nurses, and parents had little hope that they would see these young patients survive.

In a climate where childhood cancer was considered a hopeless cause, researchers and physicians at St. Jude persevered, pioneering a combination of chemotherapy, radiation and where necessary, surgery to cure young patients, then exporting their findings to doctors and scientists worldwide.

Today, cancer is still a threat to young lives, with an estimated 7,600 new cases diagnosed in the United States each year. The difference in prognosis for young cancer victims in the 1960s and those of the 1990s is in large part due to the advances made at Danny Thomas' hospital. Overall survival rates for childhood cancers have risen from less than 5 percent in 1962 to better than 60 percent in 1996. And in acute lymphocytic leukemia (ALL), the most common form of childhood cancer, St. Jude Children's Research Hospital has brought the survival rate to 73 percent, providing strong evidence that cancer can be beaten with the right treatment. These percentages translate into answered prayers. For children diagnosed with cancer, particularly those diagnosed with leukemia, there is now strong hope for survival.

Procedures developed at St. Jude appear in relevant medical textbooks and journals and are now used to treat children around the globe.

Its medical advances alone are enough to mark St. Jude Children's Research Hospital as a success story, but Danny Thomas felt his promise to St. Jude carried other obligations. Not only did Thomas want to create an institution dedicated to curing catastrophic childhood diseases, he also wanted to eliminate any financial barriers for those families who needed its help. In keeping with Danny's dream, St. Jude is open to sick children without regard to their race, religion or ability to pay. In fact, no one, not even the wealthy, can pay at St. Jude Children's Research Hospital. The only restrictions for admission are the hospital's scientific, medical requirements. Once admitted, patients are not responsible for paying the costs of their life-saving medical care.

More than 4,500 patients are followed annually at St. Jude, with approximately 150 seen at the hospital each day. Most are treated on a continuing out-patient basis as part of ongoing research programs, accounting for more than 23,000 hospital visits per year. The children who come to St. Jude Children's Research Hospital are stricken with the most devastating types of childhood diseases: acute lymphocytic leukemia, brain tumors, Hodgkin disease and other cancers. Some have even rarer childhood illnesses, like sickle cell, osteopetrosis and other hereditary diseases that defy efforts to solve their mysteries.

In 1994, Patricia Miranda, the mother of St. Jude patient Marko Miranda, said, "You will never know how much you are doing for all the mothers. . . . I can't believe there are so many good people in this world. I still have a son because of you."

Cheri Dorbritz remembered her daughter's stay at St. Jude Children's Research Hospital this way: "Our first reaction when we walked into St. Jude was one of enormous relief, relief that we wouldn't have to worry about her medical bills, and that we were finally someplace that could help her."

In 1985, Pat Patchell, one of the first patients in St. Jude's pioneering leukemia study of the 1960s and in 1996 one of St. Jude's longest disease-free survivors of childhood cancer, commented on his indebtedness to the hospital. After a moving talk about the details of his experience, he said, "I wish I could be more articulate about the way I feel about St. Jude Hospital. It's really beyond words."

William Palma, the brother of St. Jude patient Betsy Palma, wrote to Danny Thomas in 1985, saying, "I thank God for you, Danny, and all those involved who have not only helped Betsy, but all the children at St. Jude. Thank you for everything you have done and are doing. Your love, understanding and compassion are deeply appreciated."

Such feelings are typical of all who are served at St. Jude — patients, parents, and siblings. Even those who lose a child at St. Jude develop such strong bonds that they often stay in touch with the staff for years.

The amount of money needed to operate and maintain a world-class facility on the scale of St. Jude Children's Research Hospital is staggering. St. Jude's operating costs were more than $337,000 each day in 1995. That year, the normal three-year treatment for a child with standard-risk acute lympho-cytic leukemia (ALL) cost about $60,500 for the first year. The second year of treatment averages $38,000, with third year cost estimates averaging $19,000. That cost covers but one child with ALL. The expense for other types of child-hood cancer can go even higher. The medical service that St. Jude provided its patients in 1995 cost approximately $129,000 a day. And that expense was for treatment alone; millions of dollars more is needed each year for research, facil-ities, staff and equipment.

Even in its earliest years, the operating expenses for the hospital trans-lated into substantial sums money that Danny Thomas did not have. The St. Jude Hospital Foundation of California, formed by Thomas in 1951 to raise money for the hospital's construction, was not prepared to cover operating costs.

In 1957, facing the possibility that his dream might never be realized, Danny addressed the problem of how to finance the hospital's operating and maintenance. He turned to the people who shared his heritage — fellow second- and third-generation Americans descended from Arab immigrants — and asked for their help. A group of dedicated men and women responded to his request and formed the American Lebanese Syrian Associated Charities (ALSAC) for the sole purpose of raising funds to support St. Jude Children's Research Hospital. Without ALSAC, the hospital could not exist. Raising mil-lions of dollars annually through benefits and solicitation drives among Americans of all ethnic origins and religious and racial backgrounds, ALSAC now ranks among the 10 largest health-care charities in America. Hundreds of thousands of Americans of all ethnic backgrounds participate in its more than 20,000 fund-raising events annually. And, as they have since 1957, all funds raised by ALSAC solely support current and future expenses at St. Jude.

Thanks to ALSAC, no child has ever been turned away from St. Jude Children's Research Hospital because of an inability to pay for treatment. Furthermore, through its ongoing fund-raising efforts, the researchers and physicians at St. Jude are ensured the means to continue their life-saving efforts to increase young cancer victims' chances of survival. Because of ALSAC, the hospital is also able to provide for the cost of transportation, lodging and food for patients and a parent, as well as the cost of the child's medical care, thereby alleviating much of the financial trauma a family suffers when facing a diagnosis of childhood cancer.

This book tells the story of a humanitarian who would not give up, of a hospital that forged a new path for pediatric science, and of an organization unique in the annals of fund raising. It is the story of those who put no limits on dreams. It tells of devotion to a cause and compassion for mankind. It is the story of Danny Thomas, ALSAC and St. Jude Children's Research Hospital. Their story is a shining example of how committed people can change the world and leave it a better place for those who follow.

HOW IT BEGAN

Blessed is the man who knows why he was born.

— **Danny Thomas**

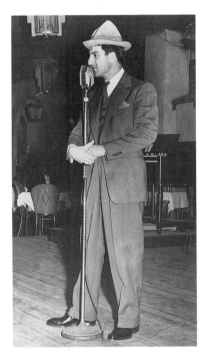

Amos Jacobs telling a Detroit audience the story of "Tony At The Baseball Game." Danny called himself a story teller rather than a comedian, but he always left his audiences roaring with laughter.

Danny Thomas liked to say that most things in his life happened through faith or by accident. Or perhaps a combination of the two. Whatever the formula, Thomas dreams, and his perseverance in pursuing those dreams, no matter the odds, also played a significant part. As a boy, Danny dreamed of making a name for himself in show business, and he devoted himself to that pursuit. What he didn't realize was how his success as an entertainer would allow him to impact the lives of children all over the world. When that became clear to him, Danny Thomas knew why God had put him on this earth.

One of nine children born to Charles and Margaret Jacobs from Becheri, Lebanon, Thomas entered the world during a blizzard in Deerfield, Michigan, on January 6, 1912, as Muzyad Yakhoob, later Anglicized to Amos Jacobs. Like most poor children of his era, Jacobs learned to pick up odd jobs wherever he could. But when at age 10 he began work as a candy butcher, selling soda pop and candy in the Empire Burlesque Theater in Toledo and idolizing the comics he saw there, his fate was sealed. He knew by the time he was 12 that show business was where he belonged. At 19, Jacobs had a regular spot on a Detroit amateur radio show called *The Happy Hour Club*. And though he received only $6 a week for his efforts, he knew that he had found his calling. It was on that show that he later met Rose Marie Cassaniti, a beautiful 14-year old singer who used Rose Marie Mantel as her professional name. Smitten, Danny always said, "She was Italian through and through, and she sang like an angel." Three years after they met, Miss Cassaniti became Mrs. Amos Jacobs.

Despite his passion for show business, in the last years of the Great Depression, his show business aspirations seemed doomed to failure. The local nightclub engagement that paid his bills was near its end and Rose Marie was due to deliver the couple's first child. With only $7.85 to his name, Jacobs did not even have enough money to pay the hospital.

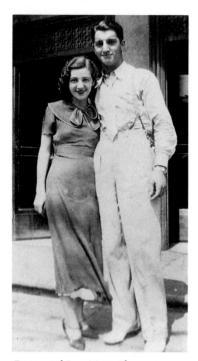

Danny and Rose Marie Thomas in front of WMBC radio, Detroit, Jan. 16, 1936 , the day after their wedding.

Deeply troubled, Jacobs went to mass. As he says in his book, *Make Room for Danny*, "My despair led me to my first exposure to the power of faith." After dropping $1.00 in the collection box, he sat in the quiet of the church, listening to the priest talk about the money needed for missionary work. "I got carried away and ended up giving my last $6.00." When he realized what he had done, "I walked up to the altar rail, got on my knees and prayed," he writes. "I said aloud, 'Look, I've given my last seven bucks. I need it back tenfold, because I got a kid on the way and I have to pay a hospital bill."

The next morning, he got a call. There was a job available — a demonstration skit for Maytag washing machines. The pay: $75. From that moment on, answered prayers became a driving force in Jacobs' life.

Still career and money problems plagued him. Instead of making his name as a character actor as he so much wanted, he worked sporadically as the master of ceremonies at what he called two-bit saloons. He landed a job here and there on Detroit-originated radio dramas, including *The Lone Ranger* and *The Green Hornet*, but nothing came his way that could support him and his family. Rose Marie urged him to be practical. Perhaps he should abandon his dreams of show business and take whatever steady work he could get.

Unable to see his way out of the rut of low-paying jobs and no recognition, he hit bottom. That's when one of the 12 apostles, St. Jude Thaddeus — the so-called "forgotten saint" and "saint of hopeless cases," who had preached the Gospel in Syria and Mesopotamia — entered his life. To Amos Jacobs, it seemed his only hope could come from this patron saint of impossible, hopeless and difficult causes. Jacobs turned to him in despair. He went to Detroit's church of St. Peter and St. Paul and prayed to St. Jude:

Help me find my place in life. Give me just a small sign of what road I must take and I'll dedicate my life to perpetuating your name.

Help me find my place in life and I will build you a shrine where the poor and the helpless and the hopeless may come for comfort and aid.

So began a lifelong association between a comedian and his patron saint, St. Jude Thaddeus, that led to the establishment of a hospital dedicated to doing what was then considered to be the impossible: curing childhood cancer.

In the summer of 1940, Jacobs left Detroit. Something inside him wouldn't let him rest; for some reason he knew he had to go to Chicago. Leaving his family with his parents in Toledo, he set out for the Windy City on nothing more than an irrepressible hunch. By the next day, he had landed two acting jobs on Chicago radio shows, with a good possibility of many more to come.

Things began looking up for Jacobs on the Chicago nightclub circuit as well. The 5100 Club, a converted automobile showroom on Chicago's north side, was hiring stand-up comics for one-week engagements at $50. Jacobs needed the extra money but was hesitant about working in saloons again after establishing himself as a Chicago radio actor. Wanting to avoid any adverse publicity from the engagement, he decided not to use his real name on the club's billboard outside. When the club's owner asked him how he wanted to be listed, he instantly combined two of his brothers' names. Amos Jacobs became Danny Thomas on August 12, 1940. Nevertheless, to his closest friends Danny was always 'Jake'. He said he could always tell when Rose Marie was peeved with him because that's when she called him "Amos" or for emphasis, "Amos Jacobs." But from that day on, the world knew him as Danny Thomas.

Three years later, his name was drawing crowds. The 5100 Club had become one of the most popular night spots in Chicago, and Danny Thomas, whose salary had risen to $500 a week, had been offered a partnership — providing he stay on as permanent master of ceremonies. The opportunity was tempting — job security, a steady paycheck, celebrity status in a familiar environment. It was a career move that would determine the course of his life, and the club's owner wanted an answer.

Thomas realized the offer would give his family the stability Rose Marie wanted so much. Yes, he thought, this was what he should do. Then he went to church the next day.

Sitting in an early mass at St. Clement's church, Thomas noticed a pamphlet in the pew in front of him. When he reached down to pick it up, he realized it was an announcement about a novena to St. Jude scheduled at the saint's national shrine — in Chicago. Thomas was dumbfounded. He had almost forgotten about his pledge made years before to build the saint a shrine. Not only did the pamphlet remind him of his promise, but it also showed him that the saint already had a small shrine dedicated to his name. Danny sensed that much more was expected of him. And a more magnificent shrine could not be built on the salary of a nightclub owner. Again Thomas prayed to St. Jude to show him the way. His answer came from a Jewish theatrical agent in town on a layover between train connections.

Abe Lastfogel, the head of the William Morris Agency in New York, one of America's leading talent agencies, had heard about Danny Thomas and wanted to meet him. He changed his travel plans in order to see Danny's show at the 5100 Club and was impressed by the young comedian. Thomas heard St. Jude responding to his prayer in Lastfogel's offer after his performance: Stay in show business and I will make you a star, the agent told him. Lastfogel was true to his word. Thomas followed him to New York, where Lastfogel booked him at the popular nightclub La Martinique. Lastfogel then landed him a regular spot on CBS' *Fanny Brice Show*, the top network radio comedy show of the day, where the entertainer garnered national exposure. Danny Thomas' star was on the rise, ultimately leading to recognition as one of America's leading entertainers and humanitarians.

But first came a detour to North Africa and Europe. As president of U.S.O. Camp Shows, Lastfogel sent Danny overseas to entertain the troops in early 1944. His performances with Marlene Dietrich helped troop morale in the combat theaters of North Africa and Italy and earned Danny the enduring affection of GIs, who remembered his visits as long as 40 years later. At the same time, CBS gave Danny his own network radio show, *The Danny Thomas Show*, which ran from 1944 to 1949. In the summer of 1945, Lastfogel gave Danny his own U.S.O. troop and sent him to the South Pacific. He was entertaining troops in the Philippines when the war ended. When he got back to Los Angeles, Abe Lastfogel told Danny he had him booked as the headliner at Chicago's Chez Paree for 17 weeks, at $3,000 a week. When Thomas returned

Danny believed St. Jude Thaddeus led him to his decision to leave Chicago and try for the big time in New York. Publicity material from the William Morris agency shows it was the right decision.

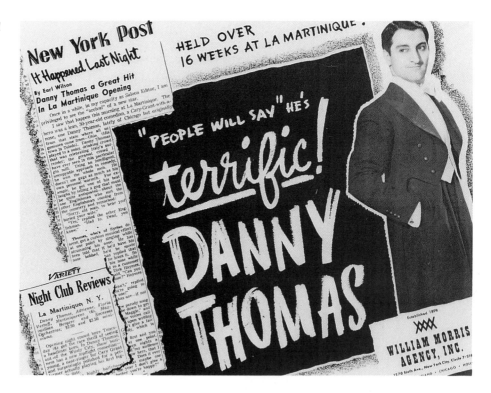

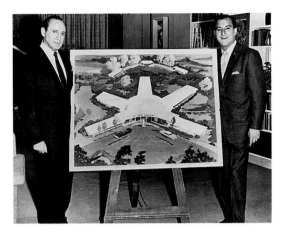

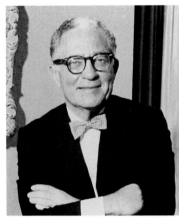

(Left) In 1951, Jack Benny, one of Danny's closest friends, was one of many show business celebrities Danny convinced to support his dream. Using only his message of hope and a rendering of St. Jude Hospital donated by Paul Williams, Danny made presentations to his Hollywood friends. It was just a coincidence that Williams, a prominent Los Angeles architect, was black and born in Memphis. Or was it?

(Right) Abe Lastfogel

to Chicago in 1945, he went back a star.

One day, shortly after his return to Chicago, Thomas visited St. Clement's church, where he had renewed his pledge to St. Jude two years before. "I lit a candle before the marble statue of St. Clement," he recalled. "And then I looked closer at the statue. My hair stood on end. What I had assumed was a statue of St. Clement wasn't at all. It was St. Jude. I was dumbfounded. It was the most awe-inspiring moment in my life.

"I started thinking about St. Jude. What he'd done for me. The vow I'd made to him in return. The time had come to fulfill it."

Danny shared his dream with Abe Lastfogel. Lastfogel had moved his offices to the West Coast, and had found roles for Thomas in Hollywood. The agent had become a close friend and mentor, and was the main reason Danny and his family moved to Beverly Hills in 1945 to pursue an increasingly productive career in radio, movies and the then brand-new medium of television. When told of Danny's promise, Lastfogel urged him to take some action to fulfill it.

At the same time, around 1950, another one of the most influential people in helping Danny formulate his plans honoring St. Jude, the Roman Catholic archbishop of Chicago also urged him to act. Danny had known Samuel Cardinal Stritch since childhood, serving as an altar boy when the cardinal was bishop of Toledo. On one of his visits to Chicago, Danny told his friend about his pledge to build a shrine to the saint. During their conversation, an idea began to take shape. The shrine would be a hospital for needy children, a place where they would be cared for regardless of race, religion or ability to pay — a hospital where no suffering child would be turned away. Cardinal Stritch told Danny the time had come to start making his promise a reality.

When Danny returned to Los Angeles with news about his plans, Lastfogel suggested they form a foundation, organize a board of directors and

Danny and friends at the 1951 Chicago premier of "I'll See You In My Dreams," the first benefit for his St. Jude Hospital Fund.

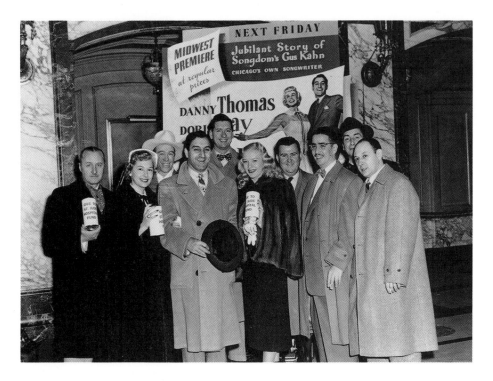

Poster for 1951 benefit in Boston. Note the lineup of celebrity performers.

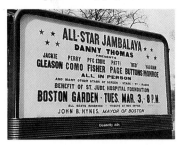

get started. In early 1951, Danny and a small group of his closest associates met in Lastfogel's office and formed the St. Jude Hospital Foundation of California, incorporating for the sole purpose of raising money for the hospital's construction. In addition to Lastfogel, Morris Stoller, controller for the William Morris Agency; Maury Foladare, Danny's press agent; attorneys Paul and Leo Ziffren; Danny's secretary, Janet Roth (Danny's personal secretary from 1947 until he died, now Rose Marie Thomas' secretary and companion); Danny's business manager, Eli Parker; and Dr. Daniel H. Levinthal were present. Along with Professor John Boles, they became the trustees of the foundation. The meeting officially marked the beginning of Danny's more than 40 years of fund raising for his dream. Janet Roth recalls that there was a sense of urgency at the meeting because Danny and "Uncle Abe", as Danny called Lastfogel, were flying to Memphis to meet with friends of Cardinal Stritch. Lastfogel felt that having an incorporated non-profit charter in hand would show their serious intent.

St. Jude Hospital Foundation of California staged its first major fund-raising event in a Chicago theater in December 1951. It was the Midwest premiere of Danny Thomas' new film *I'll See You In My Dreams*, with Doris Day. "We raised $51,000 that night in 1951," Thomas later recalled. "It's funny how that number has haunted me for years. I catapulted out of the 5100 Club in Chicago; we collected $51,000 at our first major benefit; and St. Jude Hospital is built on Highway 51 in Tennessee."

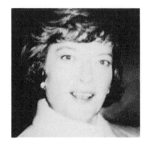

Janet Roth

Danny with his close friend and mentor, Samuel Cardinal Stritch. (Photo courtesy "The Chicago Catholic")

At the time, Danny still thought of the fulfillment of his promise in terms of a small clinic for indigent children. He projected that the hospital would cost $1 million to build and $300,000 annually to operate. As he so often told the story in later years, Danny hoped to turn hospital administration over to an order of nuns after its completion. Its location, he thought, should be rural — the bayous of Louisiana or the back country of the Mississippi River Delta, where children had little access to medical care.

Cardinal Stritch disagreed. He thought Danny should set higher goals and asked him to consider making it a larger children's hospital in Memphis. He cited Memphis' large medical community surrounding the University of Tennessee Memphis (Tennessee's only state-supported medical school at the time) and its importance as a transportation center. Then he pointed out the problems inherent in locating a hospital in a remote area. Although born in Nashville, Cardinal Stritch had many friends in Memphis — the location of his first parish — and harbored a special fondness for the river city. He told Danny he considered it his hometown. As Danny frequently and happily recounted this meeting, Cardinal Stritch took almost 30 minutes to get to this last point. "Your Eminence, if you'd said that in the first place, you could have spared me the sermon," is how Danny recalled his response.

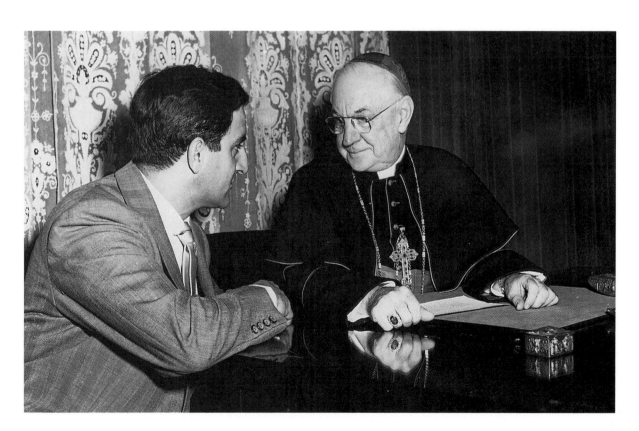

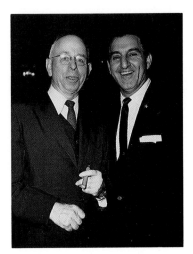

Dr. Lemuel W. Diggs and Danny Thomas, at Washington, D.C. meeting in 1962

That's all the information Danny needed to set his sights on Memphis. Consequently, two of the cardinal's Memphis friends proved to be instrumental in making the hospital a reality: John Ford Canale, a local attorney with an intimate knowledge of the administrative side of Memphis and Shelby County health care and politics, and Edward F. Barry, an attorney and board member of several Memphis hospitals who had raised millions of dollars in area hospital campaigns. Danny remembered Cardinal Stritch's words: "If Mr. Barry takes you on, you stay in Memphis, and you will build your hospital. If he says, 'No, it's too much,' you must get on your Arabian steed and go someplace else."

Barry had just agreed to help raise a million dollars to build a sizable addition to Memphis' St. Joseph Hospital when Danny Thomas contacted him. Even so, Barry, Canale, banker Willard W. Scott and Memphis newspaper columnist Paul Malloy attended a meeting with Danny and Abe Lastfogel in Memphis Mayor Frank Tobey's office to discuss locating the hospital in the city. In 1952, Barry, Malloy, Scott and Fred P. Gattas Sr. flew to Los Angeles for further discussions with Danny. By February 1955, the participants of those earlier meetings, who became known as the Memphis Steering Committee, were invited to meet with Thomas in California and begin to prepare plans for the hospital. When asked whether the people of Memphis would like the hospital in their city, Barry responded to Danny with three questions of his own: Was there a need? How will the hospital be maintained? How much money did Thomas expect them to raise from Memphis citizens?

If Memphis could raise $500,000, the St. Jude Hospital Foundation could raise $1.5 million, Danny replied. Not even he could foresee the innovative ways in which the other two questions would be resolved.

Danny's revised plan to build a general pediatric hospital was not met with much enthusiasm from the Memphis medical community. A major addition to Le Bonheur Children's Medical Center had just been completed, and that facility, paired with the pediatric wings of the other major Memphis hospitals, was enough to meet the community's needs.

Even so, discussions continued and a medical advisory committee was named in Memphis. One of the committee's members, Dr. Lemuel W. Diggs — a professor of medicine at the University of Tennessee Memphis and the head of the department of hematology and the only doctor in Memphis involved in the study of leukemia and sickle cell anemia at the time — suggested a change in the hospital's focus. Instead of treating all sick children regardless of their illness, Dr. Diggs proposed that the hospital be a research facility devoted to the study of childhood catastrophic diseases.

This simple proposal was to have a profound impact on Danny, on his supporters, on Memphis and on the entire medical world.

Dr. Diggs and the other members of the committee believed that the only way to justify a hospital being built in Memphis through funds gathered from across the country was to make the hospital a facility serving all American children. A research hospital that would share its information with other medical facilities across the United States and around the world would serve that purpose. Plus, a national research center would stimulate training in both research and clinical studies. Nowhere in the world did a children's hospital exist that was equipped to provide the care or conduct the research needed to concentrate on acute leukemia and other fatal childhood diseases.

With the adoption of this new mission, citywide attitude toward the hospital changed. Local businessmen now viewed the project with interest. A national research facility dedicated to serving children with catastrophic diseases would draw patients and staff from across the country, making it a definite asset to the city and its medical community. Memphis began to embrace the famous comedian and his dream.

Having successfully moved from the nightclub stage to Hollywood, and with his TV series *Make Room for Daddy* well into its second year, Danny Thomas had become a household word. Edward Barry capitalized on this celebrity status by planning a major fund-raiser for Memphis in May 1955. Mayor Tobey declared May 12 to May 22 Danny Thomas Week and urged Memphis citizens to "Acquaint themselves with Danny Thomas and his admirable hopes and dreams for St. Jude Hospital." The entertainer planned a two-week visit to the city to introduce Memphians to his plans and invite them to help him fulfill his dream.

A luncheon sponsored by the Memphis Lebanese community and a dinner sponsored by the Knights of Columbus kicked off the week. That dinner brought the first major individual gift in Memphis to the hospital with a pledge of $2,000 from businessman Nat Buring.

For the night of May 27, an outdoor benefit was planned in Crump Stadium with admission on a "give what you can" basis. Fifteen thousand people packed the stadium to be entertained by such stars as Dinah Shore, Carmen Cavallaro, the Skylarks, dancers Darvas and Julia, singer Frank Parker and actor Rusty Hamer (who was then starring with Thomas in *Make Room for Daddy*), all of whom donated their time.

Others who participated in the concert also donated their time and talents. The Memphis Federation of Musicians furnished a concert orchestra

Danny and Elvis Presley at 1955 benefit for St. Jude Hospital in Memphis ' Crump Stadium.

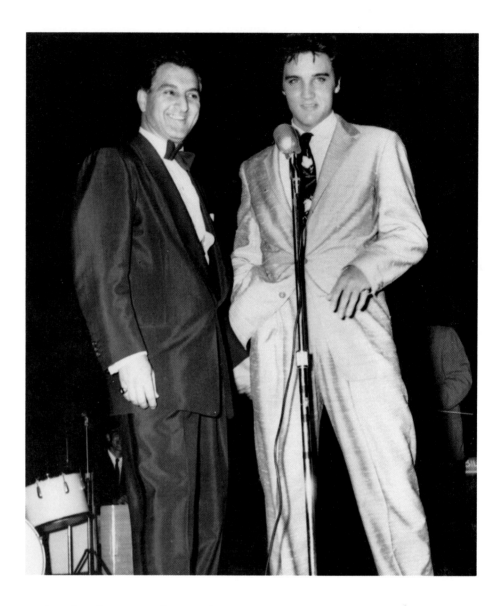

under the direction of Memphian Noel Gilbert. Workers from the Park Commission constructed the stage. The ushers were all volunteers. The local Coca-Cola distributor provided the sound system.

While preparations were being made for this benefit, Danny flew to New York to appear on Bert Parks' television game show, *Break the Bank*. On the Sunday evening show, he asked each healthy child in the television audience to break his or her piggy bank and send just one dollar to help him with his hospital. The Memphis post office was inundated with mail, and when Danny got off the plane upon his return to the city, his pockets were bulging with dollar bills people in New York, in the airport and on the plane had pressed upon him.

And the contributions kept flowing in. Fifteen meter readers from the

Memphis power company turned over their $500 party fund to St. Jude. Sailors and Marines at the Memphis Naval Air Station took up a collection and gave $2,000 to the fund in honor of Danny and his U.S.O. tours. Danny thanked the servicemen personally, promising to tell America how "you fellows who are serving your country for peanuts dug deep to give to a hospital for underprivileged children."

That spring stay in Memphis in 1955 began a Memphis fund-raising tradition for St. Jude Hospital that over the years has resulted in the donation of millions of dollars. It also secured Danny Thomas a place for himself and his dream in the hearts of Memphians. One incident, in particular, illustrates the innate sense of timing and ability to capitalize on events of the moment that served Danny so well. When he arrived for the all-star show, Danny learned that all east-west streets in Memphis had been renamed avenues, thus making the famous birthplace of the blues 'Beale Avenue' instead of Beale Street. Overnight, he wrote a blues song, "Bring Back My Beale Street," and introduced it at the show. Thomas often said that before the show was over, the city council met in the audience and rescinded the order for Beale. Mayor Tobey walked on stage to make the announcement that it was Beale Street once again. Danny recorded the song, and it was put on 2,000 juke boxes nationwide with a sticker stating that its proceeds were to be donated to St. Jude.

Never one to stand back and let others do the work, Danny gave of himself wholeheartedly in the effort to realize his dream, contributing his talents, time and money. Another commercial venture that Danny used as a fund raising tool was acting as spokesman for Maxwell House coffee. For years Danny's Maxwell House fee and those he earned for his Norelco Coffee Maker spots and many other commercials, amounting to millions of dollars, were donated to St. Jude.

Early in 1957, with more than $1.5 million in the bank earmarked for the construction of St. Jude Children's Research Hospital, Ed Barry again asked Danny the question that had been posed two years before: How did the hospital plan to meet its operating expenses? Afraid that ultimately they would be saddled with the responsibility of maintaining the hospital, Memphis leaders had asked the Memphis Steering Committee for clarification. Responding to their concerns, Barry suggested that Thomas should rethink the idea of providing free medical care, and perhaps instead offer care to the patients at the lowest cost possible.

Danny said no. He pledged that he care would be accessible to all children, regardless of their ability to pay — a promise that he not only fulfilled,

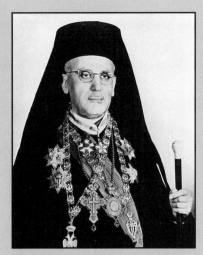

Metropolitan Antony Bashir, Archbishop of the Antiochian Orthodox Christian Archdiocese of North America from 1936 to 1966. (Photo courtesy of the archdiocese.)

Board member George Elias remembers Danny Thomas as saying, "Without the Orthodox, St. Jude would not have been built." In the 1950s, according to board member Albert Joseph, the two most important Arab Americans in the country were Danny Thomas and Metropolitan Antony Bashir. At that time, when most Arabic-speaking immigrants were Christians from Lebanon and Syria, the majority of them and their descendents were Orthodox. Metropolitan Antony was the senior Orthodox cleric in America, and his spiritual authority governed every Antiochian Orthodox Church in America.

Danny went to the 1957 Antiochian Orthodox convention in San Francisco and asked Metropolitan Antony for his support of St. Jude Hospital. In addition to attending the first organizational meetings of ALSAC, Metropolitan Antony sent a letter to every Antiochian Orthodox parish in America urging all Orthodox Christians to support Danny's cause. Al Joseph believes that this is why Mike Tamer was able to organize so many ALSAC chapters so rapidly in 1957. Metropolitan Antony was named as one of the three honorary presidents of ALSAC at its formation in Chicago in 1957.

In recognition of their influence and role in helping him establish St. Jude Children s Research Hospital, Danny Thomas dedicated the new nursing wing of the hospital to Samuel Cardinal Stritch and Metropolitan Antony on Oct. 27, 1966.

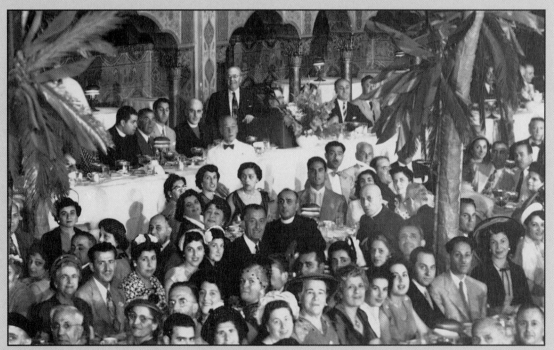

Danny Thomas sits to the right of Metropolitan Antony Bashir at the head table of the 7th Annual Convention of the Antiochian Orthodox Diocese of North America at the Coconut Grove Ambassador Hotel in Los Angeles, Aug. 24, 1952. (Photo provided by Ruth Ann Skaff.)

but that has continued to be honored to the present. Furthermore, he insisted that, by the fall of that year, he would have the means to cover the hospital's operating budget. From that promise grew the American Lebanese Syrian Associated Charities, ALSAC — destined to become one of the most successful fund-raising organizations in American history.

Danny's pride and dedication to his heritage were well-known. He had been named Lebanese American of the Century by Syrian-Lebanese Americans for his success in the theatrical business and his pride in his heritage. However, Danny felt that this was not reason enough to receive such an honor. He believed that his fellow second- and third-generation Arab Americans — sons and daughters of immigrants who had come to this new world seeking a better life for themselves and their families — deserved more for their recognition of him. Moreover, he believed he knew how he could honor them in return. He would unite his brethren in support of a single cause: providing the funds necessary to maintain St. Jude Hospital.

Danny told the leaders of Arab-American organizations across the country: "What I want to see is something in which we can all take part, because in helping children we reaffirm man's faith in man and only when that is done can we possibly reaffirm man's faith in God. Further, we would be repaying this great nation for the freedom it gave our parents and grandparents."

Approximately 3 million Arab Americans compose our nation's least-known ethnic group. Their fathers and mothers were mostly industrious Christians with easily Anglicized names. Most were from what is today Lebanon, but in the late 19th century was a part of the Ottoman Empire's Syrian province. At that time it became known that great opportunities existed in the United States, and Arabs from Ottoman Syria, including Mt. Lebanon, left their villages to improve their economic situation. Almost all were Roman Catholics of the Maronite or Melkite rite, or Orthodox Christians, all of whom quickly adopted American ways. This immigration was also stimulated when the Ottoman Empire ended age-old tax and military exemptions that had been granted to Christians. Lebanese immigrated to the United States, Australia and other countries for freedom, opportunity and to avoid oppression. The largest number arrived in America between 1895 and 1914, but they numbered far fewer than immigrants arriving from other countries at that same time.

These immigrants came with a strong sense of traditional values and roots. They had a sense of personal worth and worked hard in their adopted homeland, many as pack peddlers, to establish themselves and open small businesses. Traditionally they had incredible competence to get things done. As

ALSAC-St. Jude board member Peter Decker put it, "their love of God and strength of heart took root in American soil."

Americans of Danny's heritage living coast to coast had a variety of ethnic social clubs that occasionally raised funds for local, regional and national charities, but they had never been united in support of a single effort. In the spring of 1957, Danny talked to a dozen or more Arab-American community leaders from across the country and set up a luncheon meeting at the Sheraton Park Hotel in Washington, D.C. Danny showed the group the architect's rendering of St. Jude Children's Research Hospital donated by noted black architect Paul Williams. He explained that he had most of the money needed to build a research hospital serving all children suffering from catastrophic diseases, regardless of their race or religion, at no cost to the child's family. But he had hit a snag: he still needed an organization that would assure the funds needed for the hospital's day-to-day operation.

Danny said that by maintaining this hospital, Americans of Syrian-Lebanese descent could join together for the first time and honor their parents who had come to the United States seeking a brighter future for themselves and their children. By providing this support, his people could express their deep appreciation to their parents who had immigrated here, and to the country that had bestowed upon them so many opportunities for a better life. They could say thank you by taking care of America's sickest children. Through their efforts, America's youngest cancer victims would be assured a place to go for treatment, regardless of their economic status — a facility dedicated not only to treatment but to finding a cure and preventing for this deadly scourge.

Would they, he asked, in the name of their forefathers, commit themselves to raising approximately $300,000 a year to meet the hospital's operating expenses?

For Michael F. Tamer, president of the Midwest Federation of Syrian Lebanese American Clubs, the answer was yes. After the luncheon, Thomas met privately with Tamer and asked him to spearhead the project. It would be Tamer's job to see that the idea caught hold. Danny and Tamer named a small executive committee that held an informal meeting at the Continental Hotel, Tuesday, June 2, 1957, in Indianapolis. The 17 attending formulated a more detailed plan, then invited 100 representatives of Arab-American communities across the nation to attend an organizational meeting to be held in October.

On October 9, 1957, the first meeting of what on that day became the American Lebanese Syrian Associated Charities was held in Chicago's Morrison Hotel. The audience listened as Dr. Lemuel W. Diggs outlined the

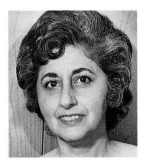

LaVonne Rashid

features and mission of the proposed hospital and Danny spoke of his plans and dreams. A program was developed for organizing a nationwide network of supporting chapters.

Danny read the goals he had written for ALSAC which were then adopted as the preamble to the organization's constitution and by-laws. The preamble captured the true spirit of the new organization: "Therefore: we who are proud of our heritage. . .have formed a non-profit, non-sectarian, charitable corporation titled ALSAC. . .dedicated to the parable of the Good Samaritan, to love and care for our neighbor, regardless of color or creed."

The hand-written minutes of that organizational meeting record that Danny also coined the phrase Aiding Leukemia Stricken American Children that day so their fund raising would have a universal appeal. The next day, the group unanimously adopted St. Jude Hospital as its official project. Officers were elected, with Danny Thomas as president, and Tamer was named ALSAC's first National Executive Director.

That evening, Danny and a small group met in the home of one of his old Chicago friends, Sam J. Saad, and drew up the Articles of Incorporation listing Sidney J. Be-hannesey, James Haboush, Sam J. Saad, Joseph R. Shaker and Danny as the incorporators who signed the form on October 10, with Danny, Mike Tamer, John Sakakini, Joseph G. Rashid and James Haboush as the first five-man board of directors. Although notarized on October 10, the articles were not processed by the State of Illinois immediately, thus creating some small confusion about ALSAC's birthday. ALSAC now uses the day it officially became a non-profit corporation, November 1, 1957, as its anniversary.

Mike Tamer was the driving force who persuaded most of the early members of ALSAC to take on the challenge of funding the new hospital. As the first executive director, he agreed to take a year off from his wholesale tobacco and candy business in Indianapolis and devote it to the organization at his own expense. A true inspiration to those around him, Tamer was known for his strong personal magnetism and devotion to his convictions, characteristics that encouraged others to go the extra mile.

The combined enthusiasm and charisma of Thomas and Tamer convinced other Arab Americans that they were an important ethnic group in America with a great deal to contribute to this country, and an obligation to honor their forebears who had struggled to succeed. As Thomas repeated over and over again, "By our deeds they shall be known."

ALSAC's first offices were located at the site of Tamer's wholesale business. LaVonne Rashid, a friend of Mike Tamer, had also made a vow to St. Jude, and felt that she could fulfill it by volunteering to help Tamer with the fledgling organization full time for a year. Mike told her his agreement with Danny was simple. All we want to do is raise $500,000 and then somebody else will take over, he said. Both stayed more than 15 years. Like Mike, her first year was without pay.

Elected recording secretary of ALSAC, LaVonne and Mike were both voting members of the Board of Directors from the start, unlike successors who as full-time employees were made ex-officio members. In regard to the files of early minutes, she says, "Look at what they're written on. We used the back of Mike's old correspondence, onion skin, anything we could get because we didn't have any money for supplies then. Our first office was a six-by-six foot space in Mike's building with some furniture, a typewriter and some file cabinets we got donated."

The first mailings from the ALSAC office asked each Arab American to contribute $5; life memberships in the organization were available for $100. There were no funds for operating expenses in those early days, so LaVonne used every method conceivable to save money. Incoming letters were recycled and used as stationery for the office, with carbons of correspondence printed on their backs. The first ALSAC newsletter was printed on a donated ditto machine and assembled by LaVonne, Mike, Mike's wife Marie, and LaVonne's mother, Edna Maloof.

While LaVonne was appealing to Arab Americans via her used ditto machine, Mike was traveling the country imploring his people to give to St. Jude. As one of the early "believers" described it, "He persuaded the non-believers by debating the merits of St. Jude's cause amongst gatherings of our people with tears streaming down his cheeks in between the 'forever present cigar' in his mouth."

In support of his cause, Tamer appointed 10 regional directors and directed them to go out into their territories and organize new chapters of ALSAC. When Danny could take time out from his television schedule, he and Mike would hit the road together, meeting each day with a group in a different city. Thomas and Tamer spread ALSAC's message throughout the country, organizing chapters among Arab Americans and gaining support along the way. The entertainer also crisscrossed America by car accompanied by his wife, Rose Marie, talking about his dream and raising funds at meetings and benefits. The pace was so hectic that Danny and Rose Marie once visited 28 cities in 32 days.

After the business meetings were over, the poker began. Tamer and Thomas would join in these games, and in the early morning hours, Tamer

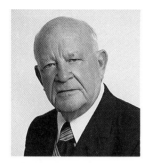

Ed Barry

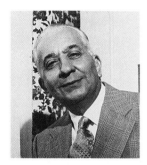

Mike Tamer

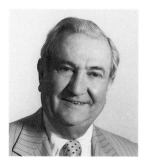

Fred P. Gattas, Sr.

would divvy up the winnings, allotting a percentage to cover some of his costs for courting perspective donors. He never once presented a voucher to ALSAC for reimbursement of his expenses. Anthony Abraham, a prominent Miami businessman who was one of the first to join ALSAC's national board, remembers those games vividly. "I don't know of any person who played in that game, over the many years, that walked out winners. Mike Tamer would cut the pot. All the money went to Saint Jude."

Although ALSAC began as an effort of Arab Americans, it soon attracted others from across ethnic lines. Even before the hospital opened, ALSAC included representatives of all religious faiths and ethnic backgrounds serving in local chapters. ALSAC welcomed anyone willing to help raise money for Danny's dream.

At ALSAC's first national convention at Chicago's Morrison Hotel in 1958, Tamer reported that he had visited 40 cities in the past year — some as many as five times. More than 142 chapters had been formed in 35 states and $159,492.17 had been raised for St. Jude Hospital.

At that same convention, an operating budget of $25,000 was allotted to Tamer for the next year, and he and LaVonne Rashid were put on the payroll as the first employees of ALSAC. On the social side, what would become an ALSAC convention tradition, one night devoted to an Arabic party, or hafleh, was not part of that first convention but was initiated the following year. Instead, at what was one of Chicago's best hotels, there was a "Cabaret Dance" evening at $3 per person. The "Grand Banquet" on Saturday night cost $8 per person.

Before the opening of the convention, Danny had asked Mike Tamer to stay on another year as national executive director. Even though it meant giving up his business, Tamer agreed to stay for "one more year." That phrase became an annual refrain that Tamer used for the next 16 years, until his death at the age of 70 in November 1974. He had pledged to see the hospital's first expansion project, a seven-story tower, completed and paid for before he retired, but he died one year before his wish was fulfilled. Without his many years of dedication to St. Jude Children's Research Hospital and his dynamic leadership of ALSAC, it's likely this wish would never have been even a possibility.

After his appointment as the full-time, paid national executive director at the convention, Tamer turned his Indianapolis tobacco and candy warehouse building into the first national offices of the ALSAC organization. For years he ran a small operation, relying on a staff composed of more volunteers than paid employees. Tamer, a self-made man with little formal education, delighted in recalling that "this man Thomas" had assured him in 1957 that the hospital was going to cost $1 million to build and $300,000 a year to operate. He would follow this statement with, "I knew I shouldn't have trusted Thomas because it cost $2 million to build and a million a year to maintain at the start — and from then on I was stuck."

When there were money problems, Danny and Mike worried them through together. Long nights were spent in Mike's hotel room as the two men tried to figure out how the hospital could afford a new piece of equipment needed by the doctors or research staff. Just when Danny thought they had come to an impasse, Mike would light a fresh cigar. By the time they finally did go to bed, Mike had found a way for the doctors to get their equipment. In Danny's words, "Mike didn't believe in begging. I learned that from Mike. He didn't beg our people — he demanded of them, that they come along and do this thing."

Meanwhile, the Memphis Steering Committee for St. Jude Hospital was forging ahead with its feasibility studies and planning, little doubting that Danny would be true to his word. Thus between 1955 and 1960, there were three separate groups involved in efforts to make St. Jude Children's Research Hospital a reality. Danny Thomas and the St. Jude Hospital Foundation of California were raising money for hospital construction. The Memphis Steering Committee (composed of Ed Barry, John Ford Canale, Fred P. Gattas, Sr., W. W. Scott, John T. Dwyer, and George Sisler, along with honorary members Dr. Ralph O. Rychener, Nat Buring, Paul Malloy and Mayor Frank Tobey) was raising Memphis' share of construction funds, as well as selecting the site and supervising construction plans. And ALSAC was raising funds for the operation and maintenance of the hospital.

It was agreed that the hospital should be located near the Memphis medical center and the University of Tennessee Memphis medical school, preferably close to St. Joseph Hospital. Memphis Steering Committee members Ed Barry and John Ford Canale had hoped that the Sisters of St. Francis, who owned and operated St. Joseph, could serve as administrators for St. Jude as well, without influencing the non-sectarian nature of the new hospital. Danny endorsed the idea and discussions began with the sisters in Memphis and the mother house in Mishawaka, Indiana, culminating in the appointment of Sister Henrita as administrator at ALSAC's third national convention in 1960.

On November 2, 1958, seven years after Thomas had launched his fund-raising campaign for the construction of his "shrine to St. Jude," ground breaking ceremonies were held on a 17-acre site using a specially constructed spade blessed in accordance with Orthodox Christian, Roman Catholic, Protestant and Jewish beliefs. The land, located adjacent to St. Joseph Hospital, was bought for $132,118, a bargain sale price for land that had been cleared as part of an urban renewal project. In June 1960, the construction contract was awarded to Southern Builders of Memphis for just under $2.5 million. Harry Bloomfield of Memphis was the contractor.

In 1959, the ALSAC Board felt the time had come to establish the hospital as a separate organization. Mike Tamer called for a meeting in Chicago at which the constitution and by-laws of St. Jude Hospital, as the hospital was originally named when it was incorporated, were determined. Ed Barry was appointed to be the first chairman of the new Board of Governors, with the members of the Memphis Steering Committee to be the six Shelby County representatives. The hospital Board of Governors was to consist of nine members from ALSAC, six from the St. Jude Hospital Foundation of California, six from Shelby County (the Memphis Steering Committee), two from the Shelby County Medical Association and two from the Order of the Sisters of St. Francis. Each group would appoint its own representatives to serve on the hospital's Executive Committee. On July 18, 1959, St. Jude Hospital was incorporated as a Tennessee corporation.

Each week there was a meeting of the Executive Committee, chaired by Barry. As those present at the time described it, "There was Mr. Barry managing it all." Barry not only managed the construction project, he also paid for a lot of it. The hospital's first medical director, Dr. Donald Pinkel, characterized Barry as the "Rock of Gibraltar."

"Without him, it wouldn't have gotten off the ground," said Pinkel, recalling that his paychecks and others were oftentimes Barry's personal checks. In fact, Barry co-signed a $600,000 note for the hospital's construction.

According to an ALSAC newspaper article covering a banquet given in honor of Ed Barry the night before the hospital's dedication, "Edward Francis Barry is the greatest friend St. Jude Children's Research Hospital has. It is no secret that the greatest single factor responsible for bringing to reality this great facility of mercy and hope was Mr. Barry, a prominent Memphis attorney and one of the area's most outstanding civic leaders."

"Besides his tremendous and numerous efforts on behalf of this project founded by Danny Thomas, he personally has contributed over $50,000 of his own funds, making him the largest single individual contributor. Largely because of his efforts, the City of Memphis raised nearly $800,000 earlier this year for St. Jude Children's Research Hospital."

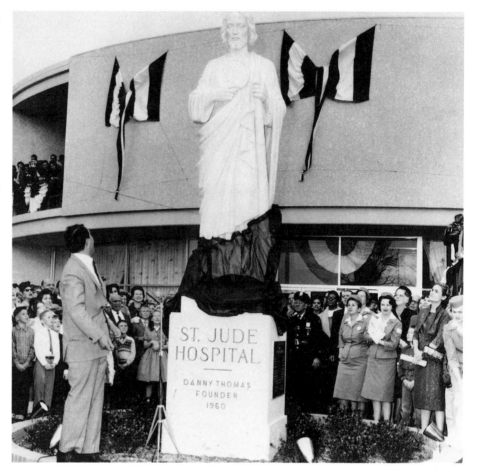

Danny Thomas unveils the statue of St. Jude Thaddeus he bought and donated to be the symbolic cornerstone of St. Jude Children's Research Hospital. The base reflects the original name of the hospital and the date it was originally expected to be completed. Due to questions about the exact route that interstate highway I-40, adjoining the hospital property, would take, there was a long delay between the Nov. 2, 1958 ground breaking ceremony and this Feb. 6, 1962 dedication and public opening of the hospital. Several uniformed Ladies of St. Jude appear in background.

Ed Barry retained his place as chairman of the Board of Governors until 1982. In his message appearing in the 1980 scientific annual report, published 25 years after he first met Danny Thomas, Barry wrote, "Maintaining a research center that does not charge for its services is a perfect example of the love and concern felt by the supporters of St. Jude Children's Research Hospital. In the final analysis, this is the main reason all of us staff, scientists, board and ALSAC are here: love, and the sharing of a dream, and for our efforts we've been rewarded a thousand times over."

St. Jude Children's Research Hospital was dedicated on February 4, 1962, before a crowd of more than 9,000. Ed Barry, Mike Tamer and Danny Thomas delivered stirring remarks. Bud Rashid remembers Ed Barry as a powerful orator, and Mike Tamer as loud, somewhat of a shouter. "He got everyone's attention," says Rashid. Danny Thomas was the dreamer and the preacher that day. A 5,000-pound, 10-foot-tall white marble statue of St. Jude Thaddeus, ordered by Danny Thomas from De Prato Statuary in Rome, Italy, and placed atop a 1,000-pound cornerstone, both gifts from Thomas, marked the entrance to the new hospital. In the cornerstone were copies of the St. Jude Hospital Foundation of California and ALSAC constitutions and newspaper articles about the hospital. Also included were a half dollar and a quarter given to Thomas by Billy Johnson, a blind and partially deaf boy from Peoria, Illinois, who had been stricken by cerebral palsy. Johnson had called out to Thomas during a fund-raising speech there, saying, "Hey, Danny Thomas. I want to help the poor sick kids," and then handed him the two coins in an envelope. Danny told people about this incident over and over in future years.

Begun as a promise to a saint by a troubled young man searching for guidance in a Detroit church, St. Jude Children's Research Hospital represented the selfless dedication of a handful of committed people and the generosity of the American public, all united across racial and religious boundaries in support of one cause. In Thomas' words that sunny but cold and windy day, the hospital was "the dream of a Catholic; designed by a Methodist-Episcopal Negro architect; built by a firm owned by a Jew; equipped and supported by volunteer Protestants, Roman and Orthodox Catholics, Jews and Moslems; staffed by Anglo-Saxons, Orientals, Negroes and many other ethnic origins — to offer hope to the world's children regardless of race, creed or economic status."

"A dream is one thing," Danny told the crowd. "A realization is something entirely separate. I publicly thank you, wherever you may be, for the support of this dream. It took a rabble-rousing, hook-nosed comedian to get your attention, but it took your hearts, loving minds and generous souls to make it come true. If I were to die this minute, I would know why I was born."

PROVIDING OVERSIGHT:
A UNIQUE BOARD

We always felt we owed something to this country, and this was an opportunity for us to give something back to the United States. Our motives were pure and very strong.

— Joseph R. Shaker

Just as it is important to understand the motivation that led Danny Thomas to become the founder, leader, patriarch and most important fund raiser for St. Jude Children's Research Hospital, the role of a small but very important group of dedicated volunteers must be considered. From the thousands who responded to Danny's call for help in 1957, there emerged a core group of devoted believers who over the years have composed the Board of Directors of ALSAC and the Board of Governors of St. Jude Children's Research Hospital. Starting with nothing, these people found the funds and guided the hospital and ALSAC through lean times and difficult decisions. Describing the board as it was when he joined it in 1966, Dr. Ed Soma says, "We were hand-to-mouth ... the hospital budget was going up 15, 20, 25 percent a year, and the fund raising wasn't." Yet with Mike Tamer and Ed Barry giving them their directions, they always found a way to succeed.

Chicago publisher Albert Joseph, who first joined ALSAC when he was a young marketing-advertising professional from Toledo, gives a very good reason for the spirit that drove them in the early year. "We were part of the general euphoria that this was one hell-of-a country to be a citizen in," Joseph says in regard to Arab Americans in the early 1950s. He speaks with pride of their role in America's World War II effort and their increasing prosperity and pride as a people afterward. Joseph says Danny captured that euphoria and inspired them. "Our attitude was, 'We can't let Danny down. We can't let our people down.' "

Jackie Dulle, vice president of research services for St. Jude Children's Research Hospital, captures the unwavering dedication of board members by commenting, "Our board members have taken on this project as a lifetime commitment, one about which they are very passionate. Some of them live and breathe the work of this hospital. And I think that in itself is remarkable."

From its beginning, the role of ALSAC's Board of Directors has been to keep the dream of St. Jude Children's Research Hospital alive. The ALSAC board members, who now also make up the hospital's Board of Governors and oversee the operations of the St. Jude Hospital Foundation in California, have been characterized as a blend of Syrian-Lebanese traditions and American generosity. Down deep in their hearts, these dedicated men and women have felt a calling to help the hospital, not only as a way to aid the smallest victims of cancer, but also because they didn't want to let Danny Thomas down.

Serving on the board is not an inexpensive proposition. With the countless hours they devote to numerous meetings without compensation, today's 55 board members spend about $15,000 of their own money attending board and committee meetings of ALSAC-St. Jude. In addition, they support and participate in both local and national fund-raising drives. Over the years, those board members who have contirbuted significant checks from their events have received the thanks of Danny Thomas or his children at the annual ALSAC-St. Jude Convention. For example, Dr. Donald Mack of Shreveport, Louisiana, presented a check for $770,145 at the 1995 convention in St. Louis, results of his 5th Annual Shreveport Dream Home event. John Bourisk, Jr., was recognized for continuing his father's events in Maine. Nonetheless, from the beginning, the greatest reward for the ALSAC board members has come from the knowledge that their group efforts were helping children live.

In the words of current ALSAC National Executive Director Richard C. Shadyac, the ALSAC-St. Jude Board "represents something special. It represents our ethnic identity. It's a contribution from us — from the Arab Americans and the Syrian-Lebanese people of America — to the world. That's what Danny intended, and that's what we the members of that board

(Left) Typical board committee meeting

(Right) Typical board meeting

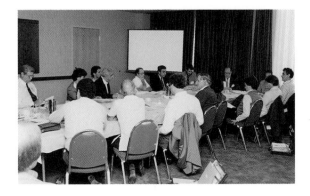
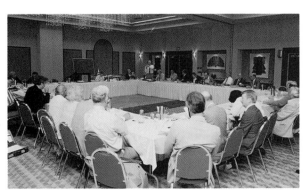

Danny gets racing instructions from starter and his wife, Rose Marie, at Indy 500 track during the 1981 ALSAC-St. Jude convention in Indianapolis.

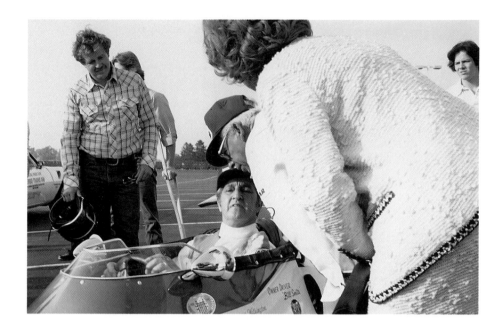

and we in ALSAC intend. That's our mark. That's giving back."

Time and again the ALSAC-St. Jude Board is described as a group that doesn't say "no." "I don't know any director (on the ALSAC-St. Jude Board) who's ever turned us down on an issue of growth or development," comments Dr. Allan Granoff, retired deputy director of St. Jude and one of the first scientists to join its staff. "They've played their role in a very effective way, and they've enabled us to accomplish what we've needed to do."

In 1957, the ALSAC Board was selected from those who attended the organizational meeting in Chicago on October 9 and 10. A general assembly that met at each annual convention after that elected succeeding members as terms expired. Officers and members could be nominated from the floor, but as a practical matter, most of the recommendations of the nominating committees were accepted.

The officers and Board of ALSAC were Americans of Lebanese and Syrian descent at the start. Members of the original St. Jude Hospital Board of Governors were a varied group of people with nine members from ALSAC and the rest of the 25 members selected from the Memphis Steering Committee, the Shelby County Medical Association, the St. Jude Hospital Foundation of California, and the Order of the Sisters of St. Francis. When the ALSAC Board of Directors and St. Jude Children's Research Hospital Board of Governors gradually merged between 1969 and 1972, ethnic diversity was introduced to the board of ALSAC. The combination of the two boards into one membership body naturally served to diversify the ALSAC board.

Today the ALSAC Board of Directors and St. Jude Children's Research Hospital's Board of Governors comprises the same individuals, but each board has different officers and separate meeting agendas. The ALSAC-St. Jude Board is composed of Orthodox Christians; Protestants; Roman, Melkite and Maronite Catholics; Jews; Muslims; blacks; whites; males and females from all over the United States. Nonetheless, the board still maintains a strong ethnic identity, with 70 percent of its members being at least of one-eighth part Lebanese, Syrian or other Arabic heritage, as mandated in the ALSAC bylaws. Some original members of ALSAC are still on the board, and there is a growing number of members who are sons and daughters of the founding members.

As ALSAC's governing body with ultimate responsibility for funding St. Jude's operation, the board establishes broad policies to meet that need. The staff at ALSAC's national executive office then develops plans and implements programs in accordance with this policy. Former ALSAC National Executive Director Baddia J. "Bud" Rashid contrasts the ALSAC-St. Jude Board to that of other institutions, stating that the relationship between the board and the national executive office has been outstanding from the very beginning. "The ALSAC national office and the board have worked hand in hand almost daily on almost all the fund-raising," says Rashid. "Our board [members] participate in fund-raising at the national level, at the local level, at the regional level, in addition to serving as members of the board," he says.

Without ALSAC, St. Jude Children's Research Hospital would be simply St. Jude Children's Hospital, if it existed at all. ALSAC has made the hospital's research focus possible. The ALSAC Board of Directors/St. Jude Board

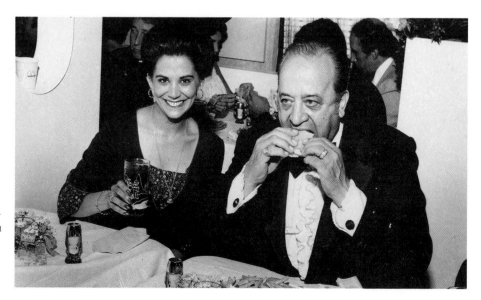

ALSAC board members dreamed up many unusual events, including this 1977 black tie dinner at a Wilkes-Barre, Pa., McDonalds. John Thomas bites into a $100 Big Mac as his niece Barbara Tayoun enjoys the ambience.

of Governors stand committed to furthering the hospital's research mission. "Our current chairman (of the St. Jude Board of Governors) Mr. [Camille] Sarrouf expresses it very well," says current St. Jude Medical Director, Dr. Arthur Nienhuis. "He says, 'We'll support anything that's going to be of benefit to our children.' " This support translates into money for needed equipment and facilities that ensure an atmosphere of top scientific investigation that in turn attracts top research scientists to St. Jude.

The board's direct and intense personal interest in both ALSAC and St. Jude Children's Research Hospital dates back to the very first year, a time that volunteers did everything. Mike Tamer's *1st Annual Report of the National Executive Director to the 1st ALSAC Convention* in Chicago, September 26-28, 1958, listed gifts received of $159,492.17 and expenses of $8,006.10, a very good dollar-raised-to-cost ratio, possible only because of ALSAC's volunteer directors and chapters.

The board appointed Al Joseph as an unpaid public relations consultant to ALSAC on June 20, 1959, and asked him to report back on October 1. In his 22-page report, Joseph called for an annual national fund drive, with subordination of chapter fund raising to this national drive. He also sounded one of the first calls for professional staff when he wrote, "But no enthusiastic amateurs — or even part-time professionals — can plan, produce and implement the carefully integrated, *continuous* (italics his) program needed by all undertakings of ALSAC's scope and types."

Joseph suggested several story lines for national publicity, including one on Danny Thomas to be titled, *From Candy Butcher to Shrine Builder.*

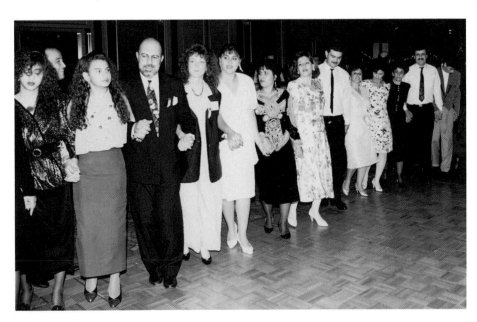

Arabic dancing and a hafleh (party) became a tradition at the second national convention. At the first convention in Chicago in 1958, the music and dancing featured American pop songs. This dabke (line dance) was at the 1991 Chicago convention.

Following this comprehensive analysis, Joseph was asked to join the board and take over as public relations committee chairman. It was also at this meeting that Mike Tamer introduced Rich White and his plan for ALSAC's first national fund-raising campaign. The 1960 drive was called "March/War On Leukemia." It became the Teen Age March the next year.

In view of the cost of fund-raising projects in 1996, it is interesting to note that at an executive committee meeting June 3, 1960, the board approved a fund-raising budget of $30,000 for the calendar year 1961 National Campaign. That year saw a proposal to change ALSAC's full corporate name to ALSAC instead of American Lebanese Syrian Associated Charities. This was proposed by the executive committee as a way to overcome some prejudice encountered by some chapters in their fund raising. It was defeated in a vote by the full board.

There were 767 accredited delegates at the 1960 convention. At the October 8, 1960, meeting of ALSAC's 3rd National Convention, Al Joseph's public relations committee report stated that one of the main objectives for the coming year 1960-1961 was to stress the "non-sectarian, non-racial aspects of St. Jude," particularly to the "American Arab community," and to enlist "non-Arabic Americans." This recognition of the need for diversity led to the rapid growth of ALSAC fund raising around the country by appealing to Americans of all backgrounds.

From the start, the Memphis Steering Committee participated in ALSAC board meetings, with Dr. Diggs proposal to bar doctors from private practice figuring as one of the board's earliest decisions. The intent was to make St. Jude different from other teaching and research institutions and keep the staff focused on work of the hospital. Before the hospital opened, the ALSAC board approved the affiliation with the University of Tennessee Memphis and provided funds to give the St. Jude medical director an endowed chair at the medical school. In addition, Dr. Diggs' sickle cell research was supported by an early ALSAC grant.

The debate over the qualifications needed for the medical directorship of St. Jude Hospital produced one of the earliest examples of the board's proclivity for fiery, emotional debates that never killed friendships. Even today, board members liken their debates to family arguments rather than the cut-and-dried discussions of most corporate board rooms. The discussion regarding the medical director had raged for many months, with opposing sides differing as to whether the person selected should be a research or clinical doctor, a hematologist or a pediatrician.

On January 4, 1961, Mike Tamer sent a letter calling for a special meeting of the executive committee to put the issue to rest. Danny Thomas couldn't attend, but he made it clear in his letter of January 24, 1961, that he thought it essential for the medical director to be a "hematologist or hematologist pediatrician" in order for him (Thomas) to garner national support for the project. In a related matter, board member Naef K. Basile, M.D., from the Cornell Medical Center in New York City, pointed out in a memo to Mike Tamer that the University of Tennessee Memphis would benefit more from association with St. Jude research than vice versa, so the future of St. Jude Hospital should be the driving concern for the board rather than the needs of UTM.

The meeting started at 3:15 p.m. one Saturday in Indianapolis and did not adjourn until 12:45 a.m. At its conclusion, the search committee was directed "to seek a physician who is in high repute in research and who has a broad pediatric background." At the meeting the next morning, Dr. James Hughes of the University of Tennessee Memphis was chosen to succeed Dr. Diggs as chairman of the director search committee. Also, the name of the institution was changed from St. Jude Hospital, under which it was incorporated on July 17, 1959, to St. Jude Children's Hospital. Not until November 9, 1966, did the board adopted the current name, St. Jude Children's Research Hospital.

Other hotly debated issues rose over the following years, but it was not until 1984 that the board would face what was then and now probably its most important decision in its history: whether to accept or reject an invitation to move the hospital to St. Louis Washington University Medical Center. Albert Joseph, chairman of the Board of Governors of the hospital at the time, says, "This was the pivotal point of our efforts, since from it came all of the directions we have taken since then. The new Danny Thomas tower, the new patient care center, the new directions in research and planning for additional new construction through the year 2015 which will enable us to embark on new expanded programs — all in Memphis — came about once we had decided to stay in Memphis.

"Reaching the decision came after the entire Memphis community business, government, medical became deeply involved in the possibility that Memphis might lose St. Jude to St. Louis," says Joseph, still a member of the board and chairman of the newly formed Long Range Planning Committee. For the first time leaders in Memphis began to see the enormous value of this institution to the city and state.

In December 1984, Dr. Joseph V. Simone, St. Jude's medical director at the time, received the invitation by telephone on a confidential basis. He contacted Richard Shadyac, who was vice chairman of the board at the time. Together they felt the offer should be considered because St. Jude was running the risk of falling behind in Memphis. The existing plant was insufficient and the hospital's relationship with the University of Tennessee had deteriorated. They talked to Danny Thomas, and Danny decided the offer should be pursued. Dr. Simone then met with the Washington University board by himself and surprised them by saying that St. Jude was looking for academic excellence and not money. "Then I showed them our [the ALSAC-St. Jude] balance sheet."

Danny, Dr. Simone and Shadyac then made a secret trip to St. Louis to meet with the chancellor of Washington University, with Danny even registering at his hotel under a false name. The St. Louis prospect was deemed of sufficient interest to pursue further. This led to subsequent meetings with an expanded group of ALSAC-St. Jude board members As often happens with big decisions, the news leaked and began to spread throughout Memphis and St. Louis. A public announcement was made in June 1985 that the invitation to move had been extended and it was being investigated. St. Jude Children's Research Hospital was considering leaving Memphis, Tennessee. In the summer of 1985, the St. Louis medical community was convinced that with all the inducements, including a major incentive offer from the State of Missouri, there was no doubt at all that St. Jude was coming to town.

On the surface, a move to St. Louis meant upgraded facilities, new fund-raising avenues and promising opportunities for collaboration with the university, its interrelated hospitals (including St. Louis Children's Hospital and the world-renowned Barnes Hospital) and the Nobel Laureates and world-class scientists there. Support from the Memphis business community had begun to wane, and the St. Louis business community had come out strongly behind the move. St. Louis seemed to offer a potentially more lucrative local fund-raising base, in addition to a possible association with a highly regarded medical center. According to Bud Rashid, who was ALSAC's national executive director at the time, "[ALSAC] felt that in our campaigns for funds nationwide, we were not getting the support from the Memphis business community that we had hoped. Secondly, we felt that being located in a prestigious medical center would give us further high exposure in our campaign for funds."

On January 28, 1986, the suddenly awakened Memphis City Council adopted a resolution characterizing St. Jude as one of the "country's foremost institutions for sick and ailing children, not only from the United States, but from around the world...[whose] many dedicated, hardworking people who have served as officials and board members have striven to maintain its excellence." The City Council, along with the mayor, resolved "to go on record as fully and totally supporting this great effort of St. Jude Children's Research Hospital and asks for the hospital's most earnest consideration to remain in Memphis, with the Council further pledging its complete cooperation in the activities of St. Jude Children's Research Hospital."

Faced with the possibility of the hospital's departure, community leaders committed themselves to convincing St. Jude that Memphis should continue to be its permanent home. Memphis Mayor Dick Hackett and Shelby County Mayor Bill Morris were "on our doorstep all the time," remembers Dr. Simone, "trying to look for opportunities to help us, publicize us. ... They went way out of their way to make us feel comfortable." (The chief executive officer of Shelby County, Tennessee, in which Memphis and six other cities are located, is called mayor.)

Both mayors traveled to Nashville to discuss the future of St. Jude with Tennessee Governor Lamar Alexander. The governor, officials from St. Jude and officials from the University of Tennessee Memphis agreed that closer ties were needed between the two institutions. It was decided that officials from St. Jude would sit on the policy committee of the medical school and assist in choosing researchers for UT's endowed scholars program. Furthermore Gov. Alexander committed $25 million to upgrade the research facilities at UTM and enhance the pediatric research faculty. Closer ties with an upgraded university offering joint appointments at the hospital and UTM was seen as a better recruitment tool for bringing in top staff to St. Jude.

Bud Rashid pinpoints one crucial factor in the board's decision to remain in Memphis: a move to St. Louis would mean the certain loss of autonomy in both the hospital's research programs and ALSAC's operations. "When you are working at a medical center of that kind," he explains, "there are rules and standards that guide all the members of that medical center, and being a member of the medical center, we would have been bound by those rules, which would have placed some restrictions on some of [our] activities."

The ALSAC-St. Jude Board has always been a strongly independent organization, whose members are emotionally committed to their mission of funding and setting policy for the hospital and ALSAC. "There were a lot of problems in terms of our autonomy — that was a very big issue," explains Dick Shadyac, a longtime volunteer board member who became ALSAC's national executive director in 1992. "And, of course, from a fund-raising standpoint, we were concerned we'd become a very small cog in a very big wheel. And we felt

... that it just wouldn't work to integrate our autonomous fund-raising principles for St. Jude Children's Research Hospital in that kind of an environment."

Another strike against the St. Louis offer was the proposed facility and site offered, which did not fit St. Jude's needs. The Memphis site, however, had room for expansion, and growth was Dr. Simone's answer to staying put. "Our thinking was that if we were going to be a Class-A major league player in the future of biomedical research, we were going to have to recruit some very good people and be able to expand some of our better programs. We had no room [in the existing facilities] to do that, so we looked at a master plan for expanding our research capabilities well into the 21st century."

In the end, at its February 1986 meeting, the ALSAC-St. Jude Board decided that St. Jude Children's Research Hospital would remain where it had been planted more than two decades before. According to longtime board member and Memphis physician Dr. Edward W. Reed, if St. Jude left Memphis, it would be like "Memphis leaving Memphis." Dr. Simone attributes the decision to two reasons: a fear that the board might lose control of the institution in the Washington University environment, and the sheer difficulty of assuring an appropriate fit after such a drastic decision. "The risks were very high and the discombobulation would be very high, and so the decision was made not to go."

Instead, plans were made to build a research tower, a new patient care facility, and ancillary buildings, along with conducting extensive renovations to bring the entire campus up to modern standards. "I think there's no question that St. Jude now has an absolute state of the art facility which will stand them in good stead for 20 to 25 years," says Dr. Simone today. The proposed construction plans required the demolition of the original building, a prospect that gave the board some concern, since everyone knew how much Danny loved it. No major decision had ever been made without Danny's approval, and board members were worried that he might object. But when they presented the plan to Danny, he never hesitated, giving it his full approval.

The professional staff of ALSAC's National Executive Office backed the expansion efforts 100 percent. "We felt ... that an expanded facility with new major research projects in new medical areas would help our fund raising, and so we were interested in seeing that expansion," says Bud Rashid. "We provided all the money for the expansion, and didn't have to borrow a penny."

The controversy surrounding the St. Louis move had another unforeseen impact. Although the ALSAC and St. Jude staff members had always been heavily involved in the Memphis community, many members of the board had become less and less visible since few of them lived in the Midsouth. Their presence had diminished to the point that most board members would fly in, attend meetings and fly home, without ever interfacing with anyone outside their circle. In the early years, Memphians like John Ford Canale, Fred P. Gattas, Sr. and Edward Barry had served as board representatives to the Memphis community, but as these men grew older and the Memphis power structure changed, the board lost touch with Memphis leaders. Once it was decided that the hospital would stay, the decision was also made that the board had to establish a higher profile and become more involved in the city. The result has been "a much greater awareness in the community of who we are and what we do and what we want to accomplish," says Dick Shadyac.

The months of discussion also led to a major increase in board committee meetings, appointment of non-board members to committees, and greatly increased demands on board members' time. Where for years the annual convention's committee meetings had begun on Thursdays in preparation for a Friday or Saturday presentation, committee members began to arrive on Wednesdays and even Tuesdays to take care of business. And committee meetings throughout the year became the norm rather than the exception, particularly for those involved with the building of the new hospital.

In summing up the accomplishments of the board, Bud Rashid says, "We have given something back to [this] country that has made a permanent mark on the medical progress here. And even though people don't recognize that that medical progress [of St. Jude Children's Research Hospital] was a result of the work of Arab Americans, we ourselves can take pride in it."

Paul Simon, who in 1992 became the first son of a board member to be elected chairman of the Board of ALSAC, has a perspective shaped by his teenage years, when he viewed Danny Thomas and members of the board as his respected elders and friends of his father, George Simon. He sees the ALSAC board system as providing a way to develop of young members through appointments to standing committees and election to successively more responsible offices, i.e. "running through the chairs."

"Still there was something awesome about being the chairman," Simon says, "knowing the tremendous responsibility entrusted to me. Yet we knew and were told that the 'first generation' had made a conscious decision about who was going to be placed in those offices. The message was clear that they were passing the torch on to us and they had made sure it would be in good hands."

"I feel that we — the sons and daughters of the founders — tagged ourselves with the 'second generation' label. The older members of the board never

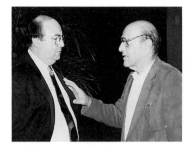

Discussions don't always end when breaks are called at board meetings. Here John Moses, left, and Al Joseph continue to discuss hospital finances while waiting for meeting to resume.

Check presentation from board member events held during the year are an important part of ALSAC conventions. Here Danny receives a check for events in Maine from board member John Bourisk, Sr., at the 1989 convention in New Orleans.

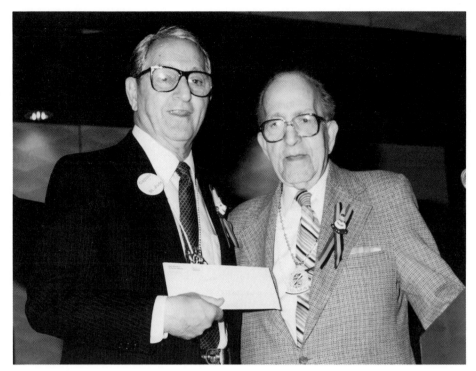

considered us anything other than equals. They had the stamp of Danny Thomas on them, and they gave me an incredible amount of love and support from day one.

"When I joined the board [in 1986] and began serving on committees I was impressed with the way Danny personally treated me as an equal, not as the founder, not as the patriarch, not as the celebrity to the young follower, but as two guys sharing a wonderful experience. He made it comfortable for me to be there."

Anthony Shaker, son of one of ALSAC's founding fathers, Chicago advertising man Joseph R. Shaker, followed Simon as Chairman of the Board of ALSAC in 1994. "I see my role as a link between the first and second generation because I have been around St. Jude board members since I was 8. I have a foot in each generation. I see a continuation of tradition, augmenting and building on their successes. It is easier for the second generation because the corner stone has been laid by the first," he says.

When describing their initial reaction to his appeal in 1957, the early followers of Danny Thomas all admit to a feeling of disbelief that a prominent celebrity could operate without some hidden agenda. They all shared the concern, "what's in it for him?" All say it was Danny's charisma and honesty that won them over.

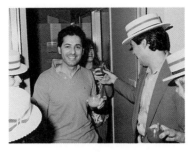

1990 Detroit convention featured loud and early wake up calls. Here Tom Abraham and his wife respond to Paul Simon and crew. What they said is not recorded.

Tony Shaker says, "Today, the motives of the first generation would be challenged. The Lebanese are by nature cautious. My father once told me, 'Only Danny Thomas could have brought Middle Eastern people together.'

"Our fathers' motives were pure. They were to help sick children, to honor their forefathers, and to thank the United States for economic success they achieved," Shaker explains. That same feeling continues, as Shaker adds, "It is essential that these motives stay unchanged. We intend to keep our motives pure."

Paul Simon reinforces that view, saying, "I view my tenure as one of accepting the passing of the torch and ensuring a long-term stability to the organization. I grew up knowing these men and women as my elders, and now they accept me as an equal. There is a uniqueness to our board that is not found at any other charity. It works more as a family than a typical charity board of directors. And that's why I was so pleased when one of our longtime board members told me, 'I feel so relieved that we can leave it now, knowing it is in good hands.' I sense that they do have a tremendous relief, a feeling among them that the institution will continue and that Danny's original goals for ALSAC and our heritage will continue."

That relief and the knowledge that the torch will continue to burn brightly was confirmed by Dr. Halim G. (Hal) Habib's comment in October 1993, when he said, "I don't think there's any greater thrill I have now, as I'm becoming less young, than to see the fact that Danny's dream is going to be carried out by so many of our second-generation people."

MEDICAL LEADERSHIP

To me, it is simply unacceptable that a child should die in the dawn of life.

— **Danny Thomas, paraphrasing an old Arab adage**

Someday, God willing, we are going to beat all the odds and make childhood cancer a thing of the past.

— **Danny Thomas**

The direction of St. Jude Children's Research Hospital took a distinct detour from Danny Thomas' early concept of a general pediatric clinic when Dr. Lemuel Diggs suggested a research-oriented institution dedicated to studying catastrophic childhood diseases. When Thomas and the board agreed, St. Jude Hospital's mission was set; from that moment on every decision concerning the hospital's future reflected its role as a research facility.

Its choice of medical directors has served to further define and promote the hospital's orientation. Each of the hospital's four directors has possessed different strengths especially appropriate to St. Jude's goals at the time, and each has been charged with guiding a growing institution.

Dr. Donald Pinkel, like Ed Barry and Mike Tamer, was a man who seemed destined to help St. Jude. In October 1960, the board met to discuss the position of medical director. Dr. Diggs, Mike Tamer, Ed Barry, Dr. Gilbert J. Levy and Dr. Naef K. Basile composed a search committee that combed the country for a qualified hematologist or pediatrician-hematologist to fill the post. Ed Barry considered this responsibility one of the major challenges of his work. He recalled later, "Here we were. Here's a new hospital. It's going to succeed only to the extent that we can get the proper caliber of men involved in it."

The board's choice was Dr. Pinkel. At age 34 as the head of pediatrics at Roswell Park Memorial Institute in Buffalo, New York, Pinkel was already noted for his work with chemotherapy in the treatment of childhood cancer. On July 8, 1961, the board offered the position of medical director to Dr. Pinkel at a salary of $25,000. He immediately accepted. Dr. Pinkel, his wife and their

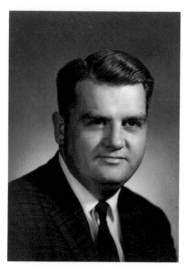

Dr. Donald Pinkel

seven children arrived in Memphis on October 28, 1961, coincidentally the Feast Day of St. Jude. Under his direction, St. Jude Hospital began making the first significant progress ever in the treatment of pediatric cancers. Danny Thomas had said that no child should die before their time, and Dr. Pinkel set out to make that philosophy a reality.

When Dr. Pinkel reported for duty on November 1, he found a shell of a building with one finished room — his office. There, with a table and chairs, plus two wires from outside utility poles — one for the telephone and one for lights and a heater — he began shaping the course of St. Jude. The Board of Governors, with the help of its Medical Advisory Committee, had set up the general framework under which the hospital would operate. It was Pinkel's job to translate these generalities into day-to-day activities. One of his first directives was to have a lasting impact on the hospital. In a letter to Ed Barry dated June 30, 1961, indicating he would accept the director's position if it were offered, Dr. Pinkel was the first to suggest that "patients be accepted without reference to financial status" to avoid the implication that they had to be poor. "I believe the principal criterion for admission should be whether St. Jude's (sic) has something to offer the particular child concerned," Pinkel explained. Amplifying Danny's original direction, the financial status of a patient and family has never been questioned as part of the admission criteria from the day the first child was admitted.

One of Dr. Pinkel's first challenges was recruiting staff. The hospital was looking for doctors trained in pediatrics and interested in researching the nature of serious childhood illnesses, with the goal in mind of treating these more effectively. The clinical research staff would see the patients on a day-to-day basis, at the same time gathering information for studies that would be used to develop new protocols and treatments. The hospital also needed biomedical research scientists in such fields as biochemistry and microbiology. These basic research staff members, some with Ph.D.s, some with M.D.s, and some with both degrees, would have little responsibility for the direct care of patients. They were to engage themselves in developing and conducting laboratory research that would help in the hospital's battle to find a cause and a cure for childhood cancers and were free to follow the research they felt important, providing it related to catastrophic illnesses.

The physicians and scientists were expected to work together, sharing information. They were also expected to work in conjunction with the staffs of other research institutions. To ensure they were not distracted, they were prohibited from engaging in private practice, unlike faculty at other research and teaching institutions.

Some of these ideas were considered quite revolutionary in the medical community at the time. Nowhere else were clinical and basic scientists working so closely on childhood diseases. But Dr. Pinkel wanted his staff to pursue areas that were reasonable and promised to be fruitful, even if that meant doing things a little differently.

Fortunately, ALSAC's guarantee of operation and maintenance funds placed St. Jude in a good bargaining position for obtaining top personnel. One of Pinkel's early recruits was Dr. Allan Granoff, who retired in 1994 after serving 32 years, including one year as interim director in 1993. Nonetheless, recruitment was not any easy task. Convincing leading basic and clinical scientists to move to the South during the early 1960s presented unique problems. Pinkel found that his best method was to convince a candidate to visit the hospital at least and get a first-hand look. After a personal tour of the facility and meetings with people associated with St. Jude, chances were far greater that the candidate would seriously consider a position there. At the end of 1962, the hospital staff numbered about 100. That figure has now grown to more than 1,800.

One hundred and twenty-six patients were admitted to St. Jude the first year it was opened. That group included children of all ages, both male and female, black and white, Catholic, Protestant and Jew, with a variety of catastrophic diseases, including muscular dystrophy, neuroblastoma, Wilms tumor, glioma, osteosarcoma and leukemia. The majority of the cancer patients had leukemia, since acute lymphocytic leukemia (ALL) is the most common childhood cancer. In 1963 and 1964, another 300 patients were added to the patient roster.

(Left) Dr. Larry Kun and team prep patient for diagnostic imaging.

(Right) Cardiopulmonary lab work is an important part of clinical research.

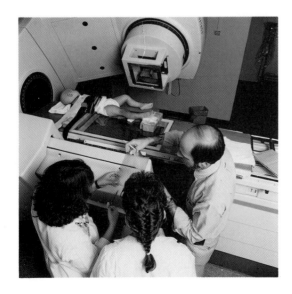

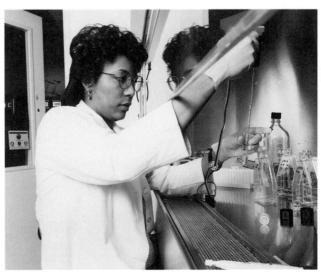

The same year as Pinkel's arrival saw the formation of another body that has helped shaped the direction of St. Jude. Created in 1961, the independent, self-perpetuating Scientific Advisory Board (SAB) is made up of nationally recognized physicians and scientists who agree to help the hospital develop medically and scientifically. The SAB meets at least once a year at the hospital to inspect the institution and confer with the clinical and scientific staffs about ongoing and potential research projects. The SAB provides a comprehensive and sometimes critical report to the Board of Directors and Governors regarding institutional policy and oversight, and advises the hospital's director on scientific policy decisions, appointments, research directions and clinical activities.

In 1965, the Scientific Advisory Board recommended that a single person should be responsible for the entire operation of the hospital. Until that time, the Sisters of St. Francis had been in charge of hospital administration under the leadership of Sister Henrita. The Board of Governors accepted the recommendation and Dr. Pinkel assumed administrative responsibility in addition to his medical and scientific supervision. The Sisters would relinquish day-to-day administration, but continue to serve the hospital in its relationship with St. Joseph and as members of the Board of Governors for several more years.

By 1966, St. Jude Children's Research Hospital was making history. In November of that year, Dr. Pinkel and his fellow clinicians, convinced that prolonged treatment was not good for children, talked with the parents of five children who were being treated for acute lymphocytic leukemia. All five were in long-term remission, the medical term that signifies complete absence of cancer cells. Pinkel proposed that they be taken off treatment and return to the hospital only for regular checkups and clinical study. This was a milestone in the treatment of leukemia at St. Jude. It marked the first time that any leukemia patient had ever been taken off treatment. One of these patients, Patrick Patchell, well remembers that day.

Diagnosed with ALL in January 1964 at the age of 11, Patchell responded quickly to treatment. After an initial two months as an in-patient, followed by radiation therapy, he began a regimen of weekly visits to St. Jude for chemotherapy that left him very nauseated. That was harder than anything else, he recalls. "That was a very trying time for me." Patchell would usually have to miss an extra day of school after his treatments because of the drugs' side effects.

When Patchell's family was approached with the option of discontinuing therapy, they were all willing to take a chance. "They [the hospital staff] had

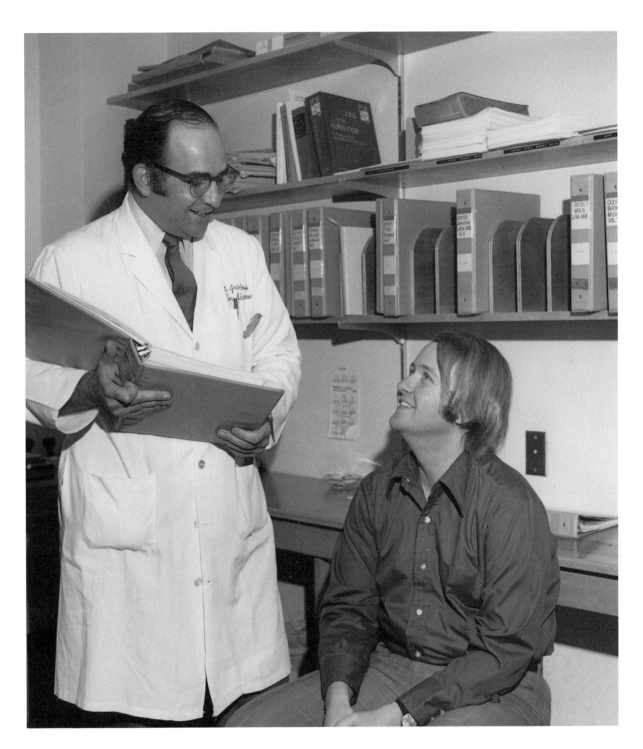

In 1968 photo, Dr. Joseph V. Simone discusses progress with Pat Patchell, one of the first St. Jude leukemia patients taken off therapy.

talked about treatment being comparable to being on a racehorse, and you don't get off a winning horse," Patchell remembers, "but we all had to get our nerve up."

After his treatments were stopped, the hospital monitored Patchell's

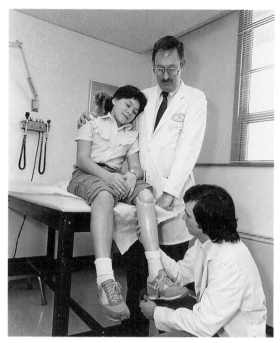

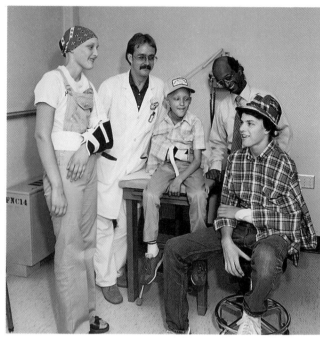

(Left) Laura Hunziker has prothesis checked by Dr. Charles Pratt and technician. Photo c. 1983.

(Right) Dr. Bhaskar N. Rao, right rear, and surgical nurse Brad Austin meet with three limb-preserving surgery patients in 1982. Dr. Rao pioneered this technique, now widely used to avoid amputation where possible.

progress carefully. "They watched me like a hawk for a while," making sure the boy's cancer did not reappear.

Patchell, who says his life today is as normal as anyone's, describes the discontinuation of therapy as "total freedom." With that move the young patient went from "some of the worst times to some of the best."

Two years later, in 1968, St. Jude was accepting more referrals of children with leukemia than any other institution in the U.S. The number of patients under study was more than 1,000, and the staff felt that they might be able to think in terms of a cure.

In May 1970, Dr. Pinkel issued a statement that would have been viewed as impossible 10 years before: "Leukemia can no longer be considered an incurable disease." St. Jude was experiencing a five-year cure rate of 50 percent for its patients. That meant that half of all children suffering from leukemia who were admitted to St. Jude were expected to survive. St. Jude pioneered the combination of chemotherapy, radiation and, where necessary, surgery to treat childhood cancers. The combined-therapy approach brought the first proof that childhood leukemia was not always incurable.

The goal of the clinical staff had been to increase the survival rate until there were no fatalities. At the same time, basic biomedical researchers in their laboratories would continue to search for a cause and cure. In less than a decade, St. Jude seemed well on its way to achieving its goal. According to Dr.

Allan Granoff, "Donald Pinkel had the vision that childhood cancer could be cured — a revolutionary thought in itself at that time — but he conceptually had the idea, and he instituted the curing of acute lymphocytic leukemia. It was that one single achievement that put us on the map and brought us the instant visibility we would never have achieved if our success had happened slowly and in a less dramatic fashion. And it was Don's idea to have an institute that would have basic scientists and clinical scientists working together to become a center of excellence for battling childhood diseases."

Focusing on pediatric leukemias, solid tumor forms of cancer and biomedical research during its first decade of existence, the hospital's curative therapies and research successes spread its fame worldwide. On the 20th anniversary of St. Jude Children's Research Hospital, Dr. Pinkel's successor, Dr. Alvin Mauer, wrote: "From the inception of its research programs, Dr. Donald Pinkel, the first medical director, insisted that a cure of childhood cancer was not only a realistic goal but the only suitable one for this institution. A revolutionary concept at the time, this guiding principle was of utmost importance in the determination of subsequent events."

According to Dr. Granoff, "Pinkel's philosophy was that we're not going for amelioration or long-term survival; we're going for a cure."

Dr. Pinkel was instrumental in initiating the successful Total Therapy Studies, a series of research protocols for acute lymphocytic leukemia developed at St. Jude that has produced significantly higher survival rates. Building on evidence that certain drugs had activity against cancer cells, Dr. Pinkel and his staff put those drugs together in multi-agent regimens and gave them systematically to patients, demonstrating that cancer could be cured in patients with acute lymphocytic leukemia. "That was an amazing advance at that time," says Dr. Arthur Nienhuis, current medical director at St. Jude. "And what's occurred in this institution is that we've built upon that foundation. All the common pediatric tumors have clearly benefitted from this systematic protocol structure to patient care. It has a dual purpose — first, to cure the patient, and second, to generate knowledge that can then be used to build for the future."

As part of the early Total Therapy Studies, Dr. Pinkel instituted the unheard of practice of radiating children's brains and spinal cords to eradicate any cancer cells that were not destroyed by chemotherapy. This was seen as a radical move at the time, but increasing survival rates soon demonstrated the efficacy of the daring approach. It is also a practice that has been carried over to other childhood cancer protocols.

In 1972, Dr. Pinkel advised the Board of Governors that he felt it was

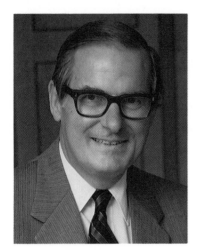

Dr. Alvin Mauer

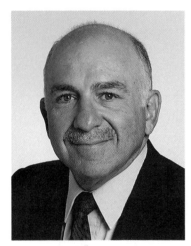

Dr. Joseph V. Simone

time for a change in St. Jude's leadership. While his record as an administrative leader was one of the most outstanding in America, he wanted to return to his first love, laboratory research, and participate in studies of solid tumors in children. Following an intensive search, the board appointed Dr. Alvin Mauer, a pediatrician who had been director of hematology at the Children's Research Foundation in Cincinnati and professor of pediatrics at the University of Cincinnati, as medical director.

The institution that Dr. Mauer took over in May 1973 had challenges far different than those Dr. Pinkel faced at the beginning of his directorship. The hospital's small, overcrowded facilities had been a source of inconvenience, but fostered a sense of camaraderie and sharing that enhanced the atmosphere at St. Jude, as everyone worked toward the common goal of curing catastrophic childhood diseases. But by the early seventies, the research and patient care had outgrown the original building and construction was begun on a $10.5 million, seven-story tower that would include two patient care floors, an auditorium and three research floors.

With the completion of the new facility, the atmosphere at St. Jude was changing. Dr. Mauer was concerned with maintaining the quality of service that St. Jude had provided since its beginning. The opening of the new research tower in 1975 doubled the hospital's floor space. St. Jude Children's Research Hospital had evolved from a small "family" institution into a much more highly structured corporate entity. "With the opportunities that our new building presents, there are also the hazards of going from a small organization to a large one," Mauer said at the time. "A very important consideration in the next few years is going to be the preservation of the sense of identity that the people here have with the hospital. We must not let it grow into some huge impersonal machine."

Dr. Mauer was determined that no matter how large the hospital grew, the balance and personal contact between the clinical and basic sciences would continue. He said that it was his intention to foster an environment where the "basic scientists and the clinical investigator are always talking and exchanging information. What we have been trying to do is build a bridge of people who are involved in clinical problems but who are also skilled laboratory scientists. We have come a long way, but we have not accomplished it fully yet."

Another major change in the mid-1970s was a move away from the hospital's emphasis on how to best deal with death and dying to the best means of promoting life and quality living. In 1962, the first patients admitted to St. Jude were expected to die. A part of their treatment was devoted to helping ease the pain, both physically and emotionally. The staff could not promise that a child would live; it could only hold out hope and the assurance that St. Jude was staffed with doctors and scientists devoted to seeking a way to making that hope a reality.

With the success of the treatments that evolved from studies conducted at St. Jude, it became apparent to the clinicians and researchers that their patients now had a chance. By 1975 the staff could offer almost half of the patients real hope for a healthy life. Dr. Mauer noted that greater hope when he said, "Our concern here at the hospital is not just for what can be done today, but what we must do so that tomorrow's care can be even better."

In 1984, the focus of St. Jude once again shifted in an effort to meet the hospital's goal of providing the finest pediatric oncological care available. Dr. Mauer, like Dr. Pinkel before him, decided to return to research and patient care after 10 years as St. Jude's medical director. Upon his resignation, Dr. Joseph V. Simone was chosen to head the hospital. Dr. Simone had spent 15 years as a faculty member at St. Jude, serving as both the head of hematology and as asso-

St. Jude nurses provide lots of TLC to the patients as this impromptu hallway visit in September 1987 shows.

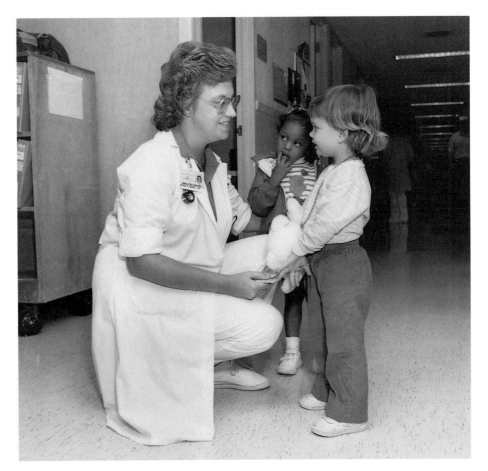

ciate director for clinical research, interrupted by a short sojourn from 1977 to 1978 as head of Stanford University's Children's Hospital.

Under Dr. Simone's direction, St. Jude's staff began concentrating on clinical and basic science investigations of childhood cancer almost exclusively and phased out St. Jude's general pediatrics program and other projects unrelated to that basic goal. St. Jude had made significant discoveries in these areas — particularly in its studies of childhood malnutrition, conducted at the hospital since the late 1960s — and had been providing general pediatric services to poor children in Memphis. The hospital was also engaged in studying childhood neuromuscular disorders. By canceling these programs on July 1, 1984, St. Jude made a commitment to focus on what it did best — researching childhood cancers and related illnesses. With that move, the hospital began expanding its investigations into the reasons why a normal cell turns into a renegade. As Dr. Simone said at the time, "We feel it may be possible to replace genes, and we intend to expand our research in this area."

The most significant achievements of Dr. Simone's tenure are pegged to his recruitment of new leaders for St. Jude. A multi-million dollar, 10-year expansion program, begun in 1987 and greatly increasing recognition for the hospital as a world leader in research were due to the caliber of St. Jude's recruits. "I recruited or promoted nine of the 12 department chairmen," Simone says. "My proudest achievement was recruiting and/or appointing these new chairmen — Chuck Sherr, Jim Ihle, Peter Doherty, Rob Webster, Peter Houghton, Bill Crist, Larry Kun, Barry Fletcher and Gerard Grosveld." Doherty, from Australia, Webster, from New Zealand, Houghton, from England, and Grosveld, from The Netherlands, illustrate the international flavor of the hospital's professional staff.

"Everything else follows," Simone continues. "The new building plan increased our recruiting ability and brought increasing recognition of the importance of St. Jude research. On the clinical side, since Bill Crist took over, 'hem/onc' (the hematology-oncology department) has a sterling publication record."

And why do people come and stay at St. Jude? Here are a few of the reasons:

I came here because I knew the diseases I was seeing as a physician were curable, yet my patients weren't being cured. I knew of the work coming out of St. Jude Hospital, and I decided I wanted to be at the place where the best results were being produced.

— Dr. Gary Dahl
Coordinator Leukemia-Lymphoma Service in 1985

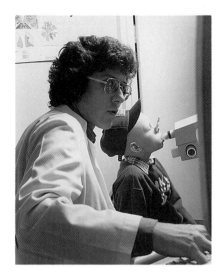

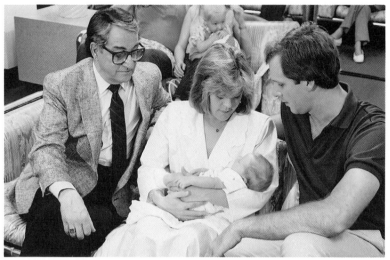

(Left) Respiratory therapist Bill Mackert tests a patient's lung function in 1987.

(Right) The youngest patient ever admitted to St. Jude, Joey DeMeo was born with acute lymphocytic leukemia and was flown to St. Jude from Florida four days later. Despite an initial remission, he relapsed and died after one year. Joey is shown here with Danny and his parents, Mr. and Mrs. Philip DeMeo.

We are providing patients and their families with hope, which I think is sometimes more important than just the treatment itself.

— Dr. Alberto Pappo
Hematologist/oncologist

The most rewarding part of my work is the patients who are cured. You have to realize that we do cure a lot of them. They are the ones who keep us going.

— Dr. Ching-Hon Pui

There are certain depressing moments associated with one's work here, but the motivation for being involved in what goes on here at St. Jude has to do with a very noble aspect of human spirit, in that you're trying to make things better.

— Dr. Geoff Kitchingman
Biomedical researcher

A child's life to me is worth more than all the gold in Ft. Knox. If I save one of them, it's worth me living. There's gratification in helping someone so worthwhile — a child who never deserved this.

Dr. William Crist

In 1981, Dr. Simone brought St. Jude into the then year-old Pediatric Oncology Group (POG), a nationwide consortium of 68 research and treatment centers. This association gave greater exposure to the important work of St. Jude's mid- and lower-level doctors and scientists, as well as that of the top

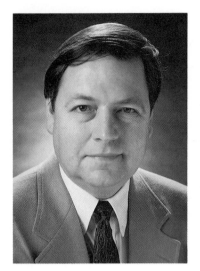

Dr. Arthur Nienhuis

faculty members. "We provided a lot of the early leadership of POG. I was vice chairman for a number of years, and at one time, St. Jude chaired most of the POG disease committees," Dr. Simone recalled.

"It is a sobering fact of modern cancer research that few institutions, working alone, can stay abreast of all important advances to ensure that patients receive the best available treatment and medical care. With the contribution of ideas, patient data and other resources to a common effort, such collaboration offers the best hope for the future." Simone notes that POG helps St. Jude by providing contact with colleagues at other institutions while at the same time benefiting from the expertise of the leading childhood cancer center's research center.

"Science changes and science moves on," Dr. Simone reflected later. "And as it moves on, if you expect to be in the forefront of research activities, you have to change with it." The leadership at St. Jude at the time not only saw that changes had to be made in the existing departments, but also realized that additional activities were necessary. The recruitment of Dr. Charles Sherr in 1983 to head the tumor cell biology department was one of those activities. "That was a conscious effort to focus research on cancer cells themselves in our basic science departments," says Dr. Simone. Sherr's many achievements while at St. Jude include election in 1995 into the exclusive National Academy of Sciences, considered to be the highest honor a working scientist can obtain.

In the following years, St. Jude's team of scientists intensified its research in basic science, tumor cell biology and genetics. The result was more knowledge about normal cell structure and growth patterns, which hospital researchers believe will lead to an understanding of how, and why, a cell becomes malignant.

Development of a research program in childhood brain tumors was also initiated at St. Jude in the mid-1980s under Dr. Larry Kun. An essential component of this is laboratory research to establish the biology of brain tumor behavior. In 1986, St. Jude was named the only National Cancer Institute-designated childhood cancer research center in the United States. By 1995, basic and clinical research included work in chemotherapy, the biochemistry of normal and cancerous cells, radiation treatment, blood diseases, resistance to therapy, viruses, hereditary diseases, influenza, and psychological effects of catastrophic illnesses.

In 1992, the leadership of the hospital changed again as Dr. Simone resigned to accept the senior medical postition with Memorial Sloan Kettering Hospital in New York City. While Dr. Allan Granoff provided the day-by-day leadership as interim director, the board conducted a year-long search for a successor to Dr. Simone. In early 1993 the board announced that Dr. Arthur Nienhuis, a prominent researcher from the National Institutes of Health, would become the fourth medical director of St. Jude Children's Research Hospital.

Dr. Nienhuis took charge in June 1993, moving to St. Jude from a post as chief of the clinical hematology branch of the National Heart, Lung and Blood Institute at the National Institutes of Health, where he helped lead the NIH's efforts to develop therapies for hematological diseases and study the regulation and formation of blood components. With the future of medicine emphasizing bone marrow transplants, gene therapy and genetic testing, the hospital needed a leader with expertise in these areas. Dr. Nienhuis had also worked to understand the genetic causes of cancer and has done considerable research on hemoglobin synthesis and potential gene therapies for disorders affecting blood cells.

In July 1993, St. Jude Children's Research Hospital founded a genetics department and appointed Dr. Gerard Grosveld of Holland as head. The department's aim is to define the genetic events underlying human malignancies and life-threatening hereditary metabolic storage disorders thereby permitting the development of specific, genetically targeted therapies. "We felt very strongly, based on what was happening in cancer science, that a strong emphasis using genetic tools and genetic science would not only be important in its own right, but was complementary to other activities in other departments," reflects Dr. Simone. "So we made a strategic decision to start a genetics department."

Building on the hospital's new emphasis on genetics, Dr. Nienhuis has taken St. Jude even further. "Never has progress in the basic sciences been more rapid, and opportunities for translating this knowledge into clinical applications are extraordinary," Nienhuis wrote in the St. Jude 1993-94 Annual Report. "Toward this end we have established a cell and gene therapy program, which brings together investigators from several departments who share the goal of developing effective treatments based on gene transfer technology."

In 1995, Dr. Nienhuis said, "Our charge is to perform biomedical research to find cures for catastrophic illnesses of childhood. In the beginning, that was focused largely around pediatric oncology because there was an opportunity there, and it was focused around the growing interest in using drugs to treat cancer." Noting that other institutions throughout the country have adopted St. Jude's approach, treating patients with protocol-structured, multi-agent chemotherapy and multi-modality treatment, he adds, "Although we want to continue that research, if we are going to have a unique mission, we have to broaden the scope of what we are doing."

In one of its most exciting new directions, St. Jude Children's Research Hospital announced in 1995 that neuroscientists James Morgan, Ph.D., and Tom Curran, Ph.D., were moving from the Roche Institute of Molecular Biology to St. Jude instead of accepting offers from such other institutions as Memorial Sloan-Kettering and Duke University. Their official opening of St. Jude's developmental neurobiology department on September 1, 1995, marked the first time St. Jude has ventured into the world of basic neuroscience research, giving it a specific research area to back up its large clinical brain tumor program. The board committed a minimum of $20 million to this program, which will employ a full-time staff of 46 and include 12 laboratories and half of the second floor of the Danny Thomas Research Tower.

The work of this new department will focus on issues such as how neurons develop, and how genes determine the development and death of different organs such as the brain. "We are asking fundamental questions of neurobiology," say Dr. Morgan, questions such as how does the brain organize during development and how do nerve cells in the brain talk to one another. Dr. Curran says, "We look at this as the language of life. Once we know the language, we can apply it to other disciplines we are working with."

According to Dr. Nienhuis, the hospital is focusing on bringing more balance to the traditional treatment modalities of chemotherapy, radiation treatment and surgery, and, even more importantly, in developing the other modalities that are now becoming available: cellular therapy, the gene therapy approach, and bone marrow transplantation. "By cell therapy, we basically mean the transplantation of cells, whether they are the patient's own cells or cells from a donor, for a therapeutic purpose," he explains, "and in some instances, the cells are genetically modified prior to the time that they are returned to the patient."

Although no incontrovertible evidence exists, Dr. Nienhuis views this general approach as having broad applicability for the treatment of cancer. "In one sense, we are like we were in the early 1960s with chemotherapy," he says. "There was a little bit of evidence that the drugs were active, but there was no evidence that they were ever going to cure patients with cancer. We were able to demonstrate that was true. Now with gene therapy and cellular therapies, the same kind of evidence [exists] that begins to give you confidence that this is an area where we can work, but we are not at the stage that we are certain of that. I hope we go through another era where those modalities will come into their own."

With its changing orientation toward cellular and gene therapy, St. Jude is also concentrating on other catastrophic illnesses in addition to childhood cancers, namely pediatric AIDS, inherited immunodeficiencies and hemoglobin disorders such as sickle cell disease and thalassemia. The hospital has also declared a goal of becoming a premier treatment and research center for brain tumors, the second most common form of cancer in children, and one that has seen relatively little treatment progress.

According to Dr. Nienhuis, "The continued health and well-being of our patients remains our first priority. Because certain of the neoplastic diseases that were once fatal are now curable, we anticipate a shift in distribution of health care delivery, with our affiliates and referring physicians becoming responsible for a larger proportion of standard protocol-based care. Our own work in the new Patient Care Center will emphasize applications of innovative and novel therapies that are targeted to patients with high risk, advanced disease."

ALSAC is the reason that St. Jude Children's Research Hospital can take up this challenge. Because of ALSAC's financial support, St. Jude's research programs are unhampered by the current medical climate. "We are willing to invest whatever it takes theoretically to find a cure for a child or a group of children with a rare or relatively common tumor," says Dr. Nienhuis. Because of ALSAC, he says, "We are totally freed from the financial constraints that would [otherwise] dictate whether a product or a given agent is developed."

As St. Jude faces the health care crisis, there is concern that the ongoing shift to managed care may impact the hospital's patient referral system, the only means by which a patient can be admitted to St. Jude. "We are pro-actively approaching health care reform with the primary aim of preserving patient access. Our unique services in providing care for children with catastrophic illnesses and support for their families will remain highly desired," says Dr. Nienhuis. St. Jude is developing relationships with managed care organizations to ensure ready access, while preserving the hospital's ability to "select among referrals those patients that are appropriate for protocol-based studies that will increase knowledge through our research activities."

St. Jude's director of international outreach, Dr. William Crist, believes that in the future, the hospital will have more interaction with its five affiliates. These hospitals have contracted with St. Jude to treat St. Jude patients using protocols developed at the Memphis facility. These patients are considered active patients of St. Jude Children's Research Hospital, and as such are not responsible for the cost of their treatment. St. Jude reimburses its affiliates for patient costs not covered by insurance. The affiliates — T. C. Thompson Children's Medical Center in Chattanooga, Tennessee; Hopital Sainte-Justine in

Montreal Canada; East Tennessee State University in Johnson City, Tennessee; St. Jude Midwest Affiliate–Methodist Hospital in Peoria, Illinois; and Schumpert Medical Center in Shreveport, Louisiana — can all treat patients of their own, but only those whose treatments and protocols originate at St. Jude through the St. Jude admission process are considered active patients of St. Jude Children's Research Hospital.

"I think the satellite arrangement we have right now with five other hospitals will change to more aligned partnerships," says Dr. Crist. "We're talking about bringing those five hospitals into a more formalized, better supported arrangement with more staff travel between St. Jude and the allied institutions and with patients receiving increased care at the satellite facility after their initial treatment at St. Jude."

Dr. Nienhuis also views the increased use of affiliates as being more efficient. "If you have a child and that child is ill, the first thing you want is for that child to get the very best care possible," he says. "But, secondly, if you have other children and you have a job, it is certainly much easier if a good part of the care can be provided in an institution that is 10 miles from your home as opposed to a city that is 500 miles away. I think we are dealing with practical realities."

According to Dr. Crist, "Increasingly, our goal is to improve those issues of quality that deal with how efficiently we deliver our health care and how convenient the service is for the patients and families. We want to meet the families' needs beyond just providing medical care for the child."

This desire to serve has led the doctors of St. Jude to take a closer look at the worldwide impact of the diseases they study, and ask themselves if they can do more.

Approximately 80 percent of children with cancer live in developing countries, where the specialized technology needed to effect cures is largely unavailable. Because St. Jude is dedicated to helping all children with catastrophic illnesses, no matter what their race, creed or nationality, the hospital has begun an international outreach program featuring staff visits to other countries, where they can touch more lives. The program, led by Dr. Crist, is based on partnerships with treatment facilities in a growing number of countries. St. Jude faculty provide support through education and training and collaborate in the development of treatment protocols tailored to local needs, resources, and disease patterns in countries such as El Salvador, Brazil, Russia, Chile, Taiwan and China. The program pairs St. Jude doctors with physicians of similar ethnicity in foreign countries for a team approach to research and

Dr. Gaston Rivera shows Danny slides from his acute lymphocytic leukemia research in August 1984.

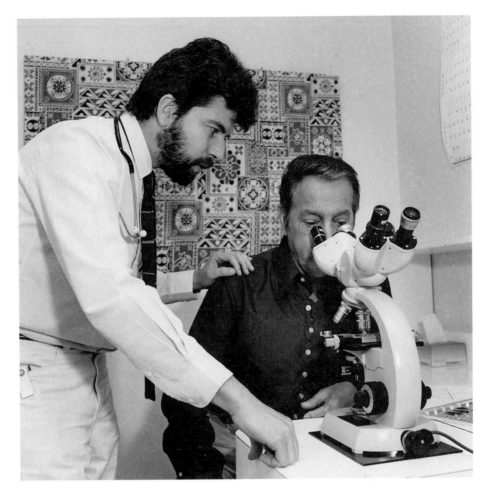

patient care. Dr. Crist says, "This is just the beginning. Five years down the road, I hope that we can document that in selected sites, the outcome of children with cancer has measurably improved, the cure rate increased. I think we are all here to serve, and the more kids we can help through this international outreach the better. It's what Danny Thomas would have liked, and that's the way I view it."

"It shouldn't matter if a child gets leukemia in Brazil or Ecuador or El Salvador or the United States," says Dr. Nienhuis. "In theory you should have the same opportunity for being cured. On the other hand, we know that we can't treat all the children of the world. We don't have the resources at the moment. So the strategy we are pursuing is to try to help in countries where there is a growing capability, where the level of sophistication in medical care is already beginning to develop, so that we can be catalytic rather than actually providing the care ourselves. (We want to) help them achieve more rapidly what they are potentially building toward, in any case. I see that role for the hospital expanding"

To assist the hospital in its international outreach efforts, ALSAC has established the position of Vice President of International Development. The first incumbent, economist Dr. Michael P. Saba, is charged with helping foreign governments and private resources develop the financial support they need to participate with St. Jude in these outreach programs. From the outset, Mike Saba has made it clear that a private-public partnership is essential in these countries, since St. Jude cannot provide financial support. The creation of PALSAC, the Palestinian Lebanese Syrian Associated Charities in Chile, modeled after ALSAC, is the first success of this new ALSAC assistance program. Composed of Chileans of Arabic-speaking descent, PALSAC is the first organization founded outside the United States with a mission of raising money to fund an institution with a program similar to St. Jude. It will specifically support the pediatric infectious diseases program and the hematology/oncology program at Calvo MacKenna Hospital in Santiago de Chile. With many years of experience in economic development in the Middle East, Saba is also investigating the expansion of the international outreach programs into Saudi Arabia and Persian Gulf countries such as Bahrain.

Dr. Nienhuis outlines several primary areas that will command the hospital's attention during the next few years. "We want to strengthen our basic science programs in areas where we can clearly identify needs. We want to increase the taking of research from the laboratory into clinical application. We want to strengthen our gene therapy, cellular therapy programs. We want to diversify the spectrum of diseases that we are actively addressing here. We want to strengthen our affiliate relationships clearly to preserve patient access and potentially expand our research base. We want to carry our impact into areas of the world where we can build on local capabilities."

The dedication to finding cures for children with catastrophic illnesses remains the hospital's greatest source of strength during these changing times, according to Nienhuis. "I think what links us is the common commitment to the child. I think the children of St. Jude are a reality to most people who work here. They see their role in life as expanded by the opportunity to serve the children. And that extends to the laboratory as well."

Danny Thomas said it a little differently in 1989. "When a child loses in the battle of life here, we all lose. Even so, our own efforts gain renewed urgency."

As longtime ALSAC-St. Jude Board member Dr. Edward Reed remarked, "I'm hoping that we'll be able to finally put ourselves out of business, find a cure. That's being very optimistic." But from the start, optimism has always been a way of life at St. Jude.

ALSAC RISING TO MEET CHALLENGES

ALSAC as our funding foundation is the origin of any good thing we are able to do. I act not as an independent person here. I act only as the agent of ALSAC, which pays the bills. I think they have a far more difficult job than I. And I want sometimes for them to come over and put on a white coat and go in and talk to some of these families in whose lives they have done so much good, because I don't think they realize what a great gift they have given.

— **Debbie Crom, Pediatric Nurse Practitioner**

When Danny Thomas founded ALSAC in 1957, he wanted to bring Americans of Lebanese and Syrian descent together not only to support the St. Jude Hospital project, but also to give something back to the United States in return for the opportunities it had given their immigrant parents. The first members of ALSAC were all of Middle Eastern heritage. Mike Tamer called upon his and Danny's people of Syrian-Lebanese ancestry to invest the time, talent and money needed to operate St. Jude. Members of this group served on the ALSAC Board of Directors and the hospital's Board of Governors, as well as serving as regional or city directors of the ALSAC chapters, all on a voluntary basis. All expenses they incurred, all travel and lodging costs, were borne by each individual member personally. For the first three years, there were only three paid employees nationwide; all money was raised by volunteers.

As the St. Jude project grew in scope and popularity, however, thousands of volunteers of diverse national origins rallied to support the hospital. Recognizing the need to reach out beyond his own ethnic community, Danny Thomas proposed and ALSAC temporarily adopted the slogan Aiding Leukemia Stricken American Children at its first organizational meeting in 1957 to acknowledge the participation of all these volunteers in what was then primarily a fight against childhood leukemia.

"Arab Americans maintained the burden for the first 10 years of our

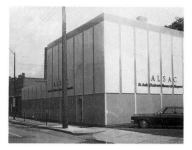

ALSAC office building in Indianapolis.

[ALSAC's] existence as a volunteer group," remembers Bud Rashid, who joined the board in 1959. "But once we became a professional organization, we came to realize that there were not enough of us in this country to continue to build. So we invited the people of other nationalities to join with us, and they did in great numbers. Some of our greatest fund-raisers are people not of Arab-American origin."

According to Rashid, ethnic diversification also meant more fund-raising opportunities. As the hospital's requirements grew, and ALSAC's financial responsibilities rose higher and higher, ALSAC's board members realized that they could not attract the kind of dollars they needed with an exclusively ethnic board, he explains. Therefore major non-Arabic business leaders in their communities were asked to join with ALSAC to foster the kind of strong nationwide representation the organization desired.

In 1957, ALSAC's mission to fund the day-to-day operations of St. Jude was seen as a challenge, but the organization's members never dreamed that their fund-raising efforts would ever exceed the projected $300,000 annually. Yet by 1962, Mike Tamer, ALSAC's first national executive director, was exhorting ALSAC members to do more. Tamer cited the hospital's budget request for its first full year of operation, 1963, which called for an expenditure of $1,428,579. In 1973, Tamer was proud to report that ALSAC's income in 1972 was up to a "new high" of $6,100,000.

In the first years, ALSAC operated with an informal budget process. Each year Tamer would announce the amount the hospital needed, and demand in his inimitable style that the General Assembly of ALSAC approve the requested funds. Then the budget battles would begin. (Danny Thomas called Tamer "the little lion" as well as "Mr. ALSAC" largely because of his booming voice and his refusal to take no for an answer.) Several ALSAC board members would always start out convinced that what Tamer was asking for was simply impossible. The funds couldn't be gotten. But the hospital was growing rapidly, and it needed the money for expanding programs and staff. In the end, ALSAC always voted according to what was best for the children, and Tamer left them at every meeting knowing they had better get to work.

Early fund raising was conducted as a grass-roots effort on the part of thousands of ALSAC volunteers and often took the form of bake sales and car washes. There were times in the early days when the hospital was unable to meet its payroll. Then Ed Barry, chairman of the hospital's Board of Governors, would sign a note to carry the hospital until the next fund-raiser would bring in the needed funds.

The Teenage Marches of the 1960s were a prime example of young people pulling together to answer ALSAC's call for help. Invented by Rich White, the first person to be employed as a fund-raiser by ALSAC, the Teenage Marches proved to be an important national fund-raising tool for ALSAC during the hospital's early years. For the initial march, White, along with a local radio station, recruited Indianapolis teens to go door to door one Sunday afternoon in September 1961. They collected $17,000 for St Jude. The march became a national event the following year, with young people in major cities all over America asking people to Aid Leukemia Stricken American Children and Danny Thomas' St. Jude Hospital. Through the Teen Marches, White demonstrated his belief that teens were basically good and only needed a challenge to rise to great heights. What greater challenge could there be than raising funds for a children's hospital? As Danny Thomas remarked, "Give the teenagers a good cause to rally around, and they'll break their backs for you."

In those early years, ALSAC not only raised the funds necessary to operate the hospital, but was also called upon to provide the funds needed to complete construction. In July 1962, ALSAC voted to assume the balance of the hospital's construction costs, more than $1 million, and repaid Ed Barry

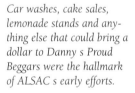

Car washes, cake sales, lemonade stands and anything else that could bring a dollar to Danny s Proud Beggars were the hallmark of ALSAC s early efforts.

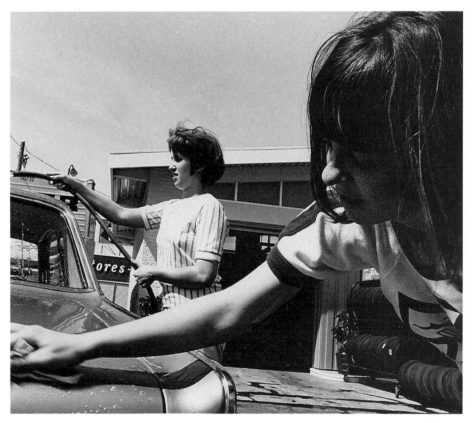

$600,000 for money he had advanced.

Often during the organization's history, money seemed to be flowing out as fast as it was coming in. During the early 1970s, the hospital's seven-story tower was under construction and increasing amounts were needed to fund hospital operation. At that time, the percentage of operating costs covered by federal grants decreased. Added strain was put on ALSAC, yet during that period there was only one year that it did not raise as much money as was needed for the operation of the hospital. Furthermore, the hospital always remained true to Danny Thomas' original intent, with no costs billed to a family for any part of a child's treatment.

Although St. Jude receives assistance from federal grants, mainly through the National Institutes of Health and the National Cancer Institute, as well as from insurance payments and investments, its primary funding comes from public contributions collected through ALSAC. Danny Thomas summed up ALSAC's guiding philosophy succinctly, saying, ALSAC will ensure "that the lights of St. Jude Children's Research Hospital will never dim . . . not so long as you and I have a breath inside us . . . and please God for that."

The challenge, however, has grown ever greater through the years, as the hospital's operating expenses mushroom and ALSAC's fund-raising goals rise to meet the burgeoning costs. The hospital's operating budget topped the million-dollar mark in 1963-1964. By 1969, operating expenses had tripled. Today, the hospital's operating budget has grown by more than 100 fold, with program expenses of more than $120 million annually. More money is spent each day at St. Jude Children's Research Hospital than its founding fathers esti-

(Left) Sammy Davis, Jr., Danny and Tennessee Ernie Ford at Shower of Stars performance.

(Right) Singer Al Green and Danny at 1980 live Memphis telethon.

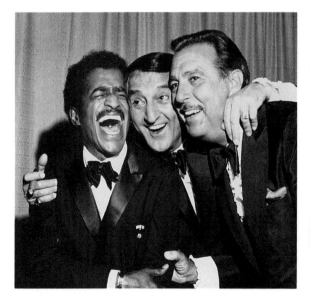

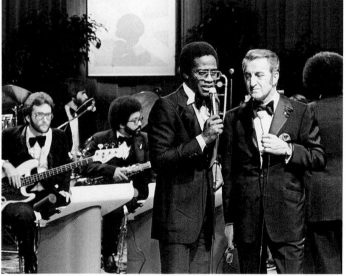

mated would be spent in a year.

Even with its success, it was apparent by the early 1970s that the hospital's growth was taxing ALSAC's abilities. The medical advances at St. Jude, particularly the dramatically increased cure rates for leukemia, encouraged people to give, but also meant ever-increasing operating costs. Tamer realized that a restructuring was in order, with more paid full-time ALSAC staff members needed to direct the work of the volunteers.

The first professional regional office of ALSAC had been set up in Memphis on the second floor of the hospital with Al Toler, a retired Marine Corps major and parent of a St. Jude patient, as Southern regional director. In 1973, Tamer transferred Toler to ALSAC's National Executive Office (NEO) in Indianapolis as his assistant. One of the first items on Toler's agenda was to reassess the ALSAC offices staffed by part-time volunteers. Many of these offices were then closed and five full-time offices were established with five full-time paid regional directors. Standards were established for the 50 to 60 certified chapters that dotted the country.

As ALSAC evolved into a professional organization, it also faced a change of leadership at its very core. After 17 years of unflagging dedication to St. Jude Children's Research Hospital, Mike Tamer died in November 1974. An emergency executive committee headed by Richard C. Shadyac, who had joined the board in 1963, was formed to supervise the day-to-day operations of the ALSAC executive office. This was followed by the appointment of Fred P. Gattas Sr., a Memphis resident who had been a member of the St. Jude Memphis Steering Committee and ALSAC from the beginning, as interim national executive director. Gattas took a six-month leave of absence from his catalog business to move to the NEO in Indianapolis. He had two objectives firmly in mind for the organization: construct a building in Memphis to house the ALSAC national office and staff and then move them to Memphis. A year later, in December 1975, Gattas saw his objectives realized.

Gattas hired Memphis CPA Dennis Morlok as ALSAC controller. One of Morlok's first tasks was to help move the NEO. Morlok, now ALSAC's senior vice president of finance, remembers, "At 611 Massachusetts Avenue (the address of the Indianapolis headquarters), all financial records were handled manually in 1975. All the membership and financial records were kept on 3x5 cards. When we moved to Memphis, we worked with the hospital's computer man, Charles Sanders, who designed the first computerized accounting system for ALSAC."

"The initial accounting records at the Memphis ALSAC NEO were kept

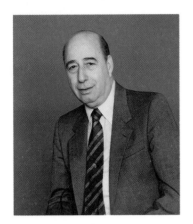

Baddia J. (Bud) Rashid

by the hospital. There were no computer records of donations [made to NEO] available." At that time, Morlok says "Ninety percent of the income was from the direct mail program" and data entry was done by another charity in Hales Corner, Wisconsin, in exchange for a one time use of the names. This procedure was soon to change.

Gattas hired Paul Parham, a retired Army lieutenant colonel, as the director of communications. Parham remembers his first day, April 1, 1976, clearly. "There were a total of nine employees at the NEO, three secretaries, two clerks and four professional staff. Fred had told me I would be doing by myself what I had eight people working on in my last Army job. That didn't faze me because it was all creative work. What he had not told me was that I would also be responsible for purchasing, printing, filming, receiving, storing and/or shipping the fund raising and public relations materials I wrote, designed and created. In those days, we were really lean and mean and everybody did two, three and four different jobs."

On July 1, 1976, Bud Rashid, director of operations of the antitrust division of the Justice Department, retired from that position and took over the helm of ALSAC, after more than 15 years of active involvement in the organization as a volunteer and board member. Under Rashid, ALSAC truly became a professional fund-raising organization and a leader among charities for its innovative and sophisticated fund-raising programs.

Rashid characterizes ALSAC's growth during his years as national executive director as "meteoric." When he took office, ALSAC was raising approximately $15 million a year — a considerable sum, but not enough to support a hospital poised for substantial growth. In order to fund St. Jude's development, ALSAC had to expand its operations tremendously, and Rashid began recruiting and expanding the professional staff of the NEO. Then he began to strengthen the staff of regional offices, bringing professionals into what had previously been mostly a volunteer structure. "With that professional staff, and with the creativity of our staff — they came up with so many new fund-raising concepts and programs — we were able to build that $15 million a year to $120 million a year by the time I left."

In conjunction with spurring the expansion of ALSAC's professional staff, Rashid was also interested in broadening the scope of ALSAC's operations. One of his first goals was to bring to ALSAC a more business-like structure by imposing centralized accounting procedures, placing tighter controls on expenses and establishing new fund-raising guidelines. For the first time, ALSAC chapters were given a fiscal procedures manual and professional instructions on how to account for money raised. His next objective was to increase ALSAC's fund-raising efforts in all parts of the U.S., since some areas of the country knew little about the hospital and its fight against catastrophic childhood diseases. Finally, he wanted to increase the fund balance to provide adequate reserves for the continued operation of the hospital in the event that economic conditions caused a decrease in fund-raising revenues.

In early 1977, Bud Rashid won the board of directors approval for his plans. William J. Kirwen was hired as director of development and charged with increasing the income from volunteer groups nationwide, assuming control of all volunteer fund-raising activities across the country. Within two months, Kirwen's Community Development Program was being tested. This innovative new fund-raiser, targeted at communities of 15,000 or less throughout the country, relied on telephones, support material and incentives to organize and conduct a once-a-year bike ride or door-to-door campaign. The fall 1977 pilot program brought in $77,000. Since then CDP has grown into a multi-million dollar telemarketing program that reaches people in more than 20,000 communities each year. In CDP, now called telemarketing by ALSAC,

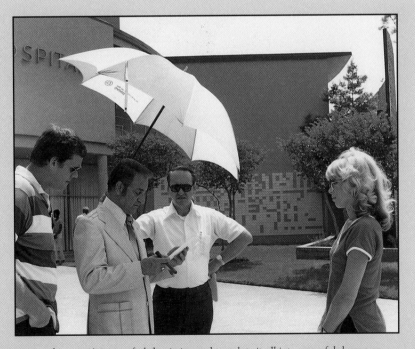

Danny reviews his lines for national public service announcements in 1981. Shelby County Sheriff's Department's Lieutenant Dave Wing at left, ALSAC director of communications Paul Parham and makeup technician Patty Miller help. A man of simple tastes, Danny shunned limos and when in Memphis used only two officers of the Sheriff's celebrity protection squad, riding as a front seat passenger in an unmarked car.

Danny's Emmy Award winning success in television, both in front of and behind the cameras, was said to come from his superb ability to rapidly learn lines, grasp the writer's intent, feel the timing and translate it all into powerful drama or high humor, whatever the script called for. At ALSAC, his taping normally consisted of one take, followed by one more for safety, because the first take of a scene was invariably perfect.

NEO carved out a market that has only lately begun to attract other charities, which historically have been more interested in major urban areas.

One of Rashid's primary goals to maintain a funding reserve equal to a full year of the hospital's operating expenses was not only met during his tenure, but has now been surpassed. It took almost 20 years for ALSAC to build its fund balances to the point where money raised in one year could be earmarked for the hospital's operating expenses in the following year. In 1983, ALSAC met Rashid's goal of having a full year's reserve of funds on hand for the first time in its history. That year, the combined fund balance at the end of fiscal year 1983 showed sufficient funds on hand to cover the entire fiscal year 1984 operating budget. This growth in the fund balance would provide St. Jude with the means to continue its life-saving research and patient care even if monetary gifts should suddenly cease. ALSAC now tries to operate with a three-year budget reserve.

Rashid's tenure also saw physical growth at St. Jude Children's Research Hospital that required additional funds from ALSAC. Nonetheless, ALSAC made history by paying for two huge expansion projects on a pay-as-you-build plan. The hospital's 1981 animal and disease confinement laboratory for infectious disease research and cancer research using small pure-bred laboratory animals and the 10-year, multimillion dollar expansion begun in 1987 were both paid for without any borrowed money. Rashid explains that this was possible because of the expanded, innovative fund-raising campaigns developed by his staff. They were doing very well, he says, "So we put some in reserve. We built a rather large reserve, and we were beginning an endowment fund, and we were also putting aside money for the expansion — all from our normal fund-raising."

Rashid retired from his position as national executive director on July 1, 1992, after serving 16 years. His leadership, foresight and planning were prime ingredients in ensuring a more secure financial future for St. Jude Children's Research Hospital, and his tenure saw ALSAC grow to a highly skilled organization ranking in the top eight of national health-care charities in terms of dollars raised.

ALSAC's responsibility to St. Jude covers all aspects of the hospital's services, including medical care — the cost of services received by patients in the treatment of their disease — clinical and laboratory research expenditures — including expenses for laboratories, technicians, supplies and salaries of personnel needed — and education, training and community services expenses, representing the costs to inform general and specialized audiences about research

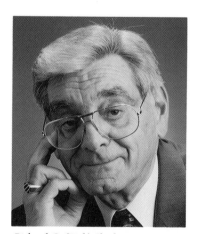

Richard C. (Dick) Shadyac

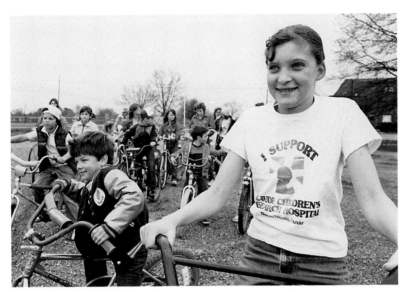

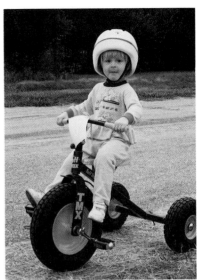

(Left) Starting point of a bike ride in 1983.

(Right) Shelby Lyn Peters, 2-1/2, rides in a Red Cloud, Neb., trike-a-thon. A spin-off of the CDP bike rides, the St. Jude trike-a-thons teach small children riding toy safety. Coordinators recruited in day care centers read a daily story of "The Adventures Of Bikewell Bear" over four days before the children ride on an enclosed course.

and treatment procedures and advances in catastrophic childhood illnesses.

Through the years, ALSAC's success in fulfilling its role of funding the hospital has been best reflected in the continual growth and progress exhibited at St. Jude. Despite the loss of its most important leader with the death of Danny Thomas in 1991, ALSAC rededicated itself to its mission and moved forward with even more ambitious objectives. Childhood cancer is a formidable adversary. In light of St. Jude's record in terms of lives saved, the people at ALSAC-St. Jude Children's Research Hospital knew that children around the world needed them to continue their work.

Richard C. Shadyac took the NEO reins from the retiring Bud Rashid in 1992. Leaving his prominent Washington, D.C., law firm, Shadyac now heads a staff of approximately 175 full-time employees nationwide who coordinate ALSAC volunteers and fund-raising programs. With one of the smallest professional staffs of all the nation's major health care charities, more than half of whom hold clerical or support positions, ALSAC may very well have the highest dollar raised per employee ratio in the fund-raising world.

The cornerstone of ALSAC's success is its strong centralized National Executive Office. At its Memphis headquarters, ALSAC's NEO staff creates and administers the programs that are responsible for placing the organization among the most successful fund-raising institutions in America. The NEO staff provides professional expertise and administrative support for fund-raising campaigns conducted throughout the country, from golf tournaments, live local telethons, walk-a-thons, dinners and auctions coordinated through the regional offices to telemarketing events such as Math-A-Thons and bike-a-thons organized through ALSAC's two Volunteer Service Centers.

ALSAC-St. Jude chapters nationwide are also overseen by the Memphis office through the regional offices. Each chapter is required to have at least one fund-raising event per year as part of its certification. A centralized accounting system ensures proper stewardship of money donated by the contributing public.

Since its formation in a Chicago hotel in 1957, ALSAC has raised more than $1 billion for St. Jude Children's Research Hospital. In its first year, the organization raised $159,492; in the fiscal year ending June 30, 1996, fund-raising revenues reached better than $175 million, the best year in ALSAC history.

Even with its flourishing fund-raising efforts, the cost of fund raising for St. Jude for years has hovered between 10 and 15 percent, one of the lowest of any national charity. From the start, ALSAC has prided itself on keeping fund-raising expenses low. An example is an April 3, 1963, note from Mike Tamer to To Whom It May Concern stating, "This will confirm that Mr. Mitchell Awn, 150 97th Street, Brooklyn, New York, in the performance of his duties as ALSAC New York State Director, through the year 1962 incurred, without recompense or reimbursement, expenses totaling $160 for traveling, organizing meetings, and conducting campaigns for our organization."

Approximately 85 percent of every dollar raised by ALSAC is applied to the current or future needs of the hospital, with around 10 percent allocated for raising additional funds and 5 percent used for administration costs. Furthermore, ALSAC has maintained exemplary relationships since 1976 with the Council of Better Business Bureau's Philanthropic Advisory Service and the National Charities Information Bureau, which serve as third-party watchdog agencies over national charities.

Nonetheless, the organization does not rest on its laurels. Fund-raising is a never-ending pursuit, with ALSAC's most productive programs running the gamut from direct mail appeals, television specials, radiothons and telemarketing to planned giving, the Combined Federal Campaign, corporate and foundation grants, memorials and endowments. Dinners, golf and tennis tournaments, and numerous other local events each year also contribute to its success.

Shadyac credits the children of St. Jude for ALSAC's phenomenal fund-raising success, along with Danny Thomas and the image he projected to the world. "His dream was about saving the lives of children, not about raising money," says Shadyac. "And that's the message that ALSAC projects. We raise a lot of money to do the work of Danny's dream, but it's the bottom line, the children. That's why we are successful."

REACHING THE WORLD WITH
RESEARCH AND EDUCATION

If you really want to invest, if you really want to get the most out of your money, invest in research. If someone discovers a new drug it can be used for decades — even centuries, maybe — and affect millions of kids. That's why St. Jude is a research institution. Although the research is done in Memphis, it applies to children all over the world.

Dr. Walter T. Hughes
Arthur Ashe Chair for Pediatric AIDS Research
at St. Jude Children's Research Hospital

A father is on the phone to St. Jude Children's Research Hospital, calling long distance. His son has been diagnosed with a soft-tissue tumor, and the man is uncertain as to what he should do. The St. Jude staff member on the line is reassuring. "I have boys your son's age," she says, "and I'll tell you what I'd do." She recommends that the boy's father ask his son's physician to call a St. Jude doctor for a consultation. "They do this all the time," she says. "There's no charge."

Shared information is the rule rather than the exception at St. Jude. Whether in the form of free written or telephone consultations or through internationally published research findings, St. Jude doctors and scientists have always believed that information about their work should be available to anyone who will benefit from it. This commitment to the accessibility of their findings has taken many forms and sent St. Jude doctors and scientists around the globe. It is an essential part of a commitment to excellence in research and education and a sharing of medical progress with the entire world that began even before the hospital opened.

One month after St. Jude Children's Research Hospital's November 1958 ground-breaking ceremony, Plough Inc., a Memphis-based drug and cosmetics firm, gave ALSAC its first research grant. The $10,000 grant was awarded to Dr. Lemuel W. Diggs for the continuation of his work on sickle cell

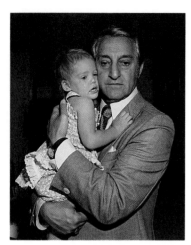

Danny with Karen Wilkerson in 1979. Karen is now a St. Jude alumna.

anemia and related studies conducted in his laboratories at the University of Tennessee Memphis. Dr. Diggs first report to ALSAC in 1959 took the form of a three-page, double-spaced typewritten paper. This was, in fact, the world's first comprehensive study of sickle cell disease and its impact on the black population of the world.

By 1962, the end of the hospital's first year of operation, more than 30 research projects had been instituted and four completed. In that first year, researchers published more than a dozen papers. Today, St. Jude faculty members author an average of more than 300 professional papers annually describing their research investigations and clinical findings.

Through the years, both clinical and basic researchers have made monumental strides in identifying and fine-tuning effective cancer therapies. St. Jude physicians and scientists combine basic biomedical research — that is, research usually done in laboratories — and clinical research — research involving patient care and treatment — in a double-barreled approach aimed at curing childhood catastrophic diseases. Once a promising treatment protocol has been developed, sometimes in collaboration with scientists from other institutions, it is tested in the hospital's clinics. Until then, its value is theoretical. Clinical testing of new treatments is the culmination of intensive efforts by researchers in a variety of disciplines.

St. Jude's research programs still follow the philosophy established more than 30 years ago by the hospital's first medical director, Dr. Donald Pinkel, who insisted that the cure of childhood cancer was not only a realistic goal, but the only suitable one for St. Jude Children's Research Hospital.

With this in mind, St. Jude researchers are directing their efforts at understanding the molecular, genetic and chemical bases of catastrophic diseases in children, identifying and testing potential cures for such diseases, and promoting their prevention. In addition to intensive clinical study in the areas of hematology, oncology, infectious diseases, neurology, child health care and behavioral medicine, St. Jude conducts research in biochemistry, virology, immunology, molecular pharmacology, pathology, pharmacological sciences, tumor cell biology, genetics, and cell and gene therapies. In essence, the work of St. Jude Children's Research Hospital seeks to solve the mysteries of catastrophic childhood diseases and learn their cause, cure and prevention, and to extend its findings throughout the medical world.

As a teaching hospital, the education and training programs of St. Jude are an essential part of its commitment to excellence. A combination of clinical and basic science investigators working closely together is perhaps the hospital's greatest training resource, permitting a variety of interdisciplinary programs for research fellows who have already earned an M.D. or Ph.D. degree and have overlapping interests in medicine and biology. Programs lasting from one to three years are available for postdoctoral fellows through a number of sources, including National Institutes of Health grant awards, the Howard Hughes Medical Institute and institutional funds. St. Jude Children's Research Hospital also sponsors a number of named fellowships: The John H. Sununu, George J. Mitchell, and Richard A. Gephardt Endowed Fellowships in Basic Research; The Morrison Fellowship; the Journey Memorial Fellowship in Biomedical Research and the Levy Fellowship in Cancer Medicine; the Karnofsky Fellowship in Cancer Research; and the Lemuel W. Diggs Fellowship in Experimental Hematology. Regardless of the program selected, trainees are given the opportunity to work closely with St. Jude senior faculty members and to attend regularly scheduled seminars, workshops, journal clubs and lectures. Other St. Jude programs offer experience and training in behavioral medicine

Danny shows his Congressional Gold Medal to a patient in April 1985. He went directly from the White House ceremony to St. Jude so he could share his recognition with those who helped him get it.

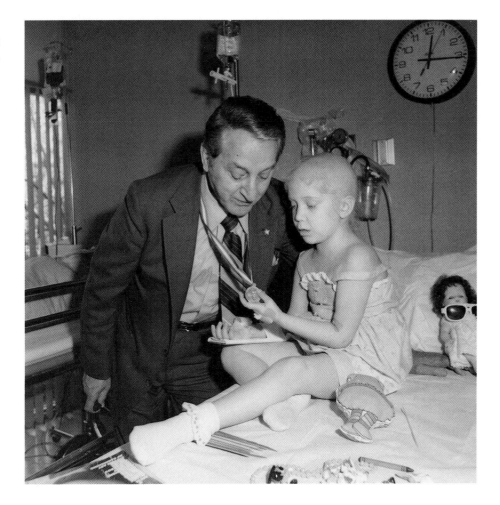

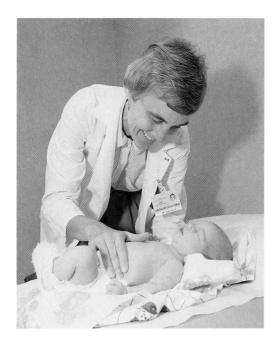

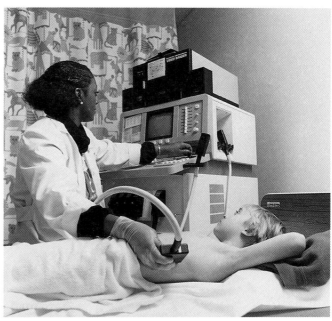

(Left) Dr. Ann Hayes with neuroblastoma patient. Dr. Hayes and Dr. Alexander Green were the St. Jude pioneers who found treatments for what was an almost uniformly fatal illness until 1976.

(Right) Mary Alice Fitzpatrick runs diagnostic imaging test on Nicholas Gentry.

and related specialties. Fellowships are available in the psychology division, and the pastoral care division has internships for seminary students. Social work programs are also available, with a training grant supporting social work internships for master's degree candidates.

Physicians, scientists and nurses from around the world travel to St. Jude for information, both to learn first-hand about the hospital's new developments and to further their own training. Young M.D.s, Ph.D.s and nurses seeking graduate training or continuing education have long looked to St. Jude Children's Research Hospital as an excellent professional training environment in which to further their education before moving on to apply their knowledge at hospitals and research centers across the nation and in some foreign countries. Moreover, each February, St. Jude hosts a two-day symposium for referring physicians to familiarize them with the center's facilities and staff and acquaint them with the latest methods employed for the cure and treatment of childhood cancers and other life-threatening diseases.

In 1988, the Fellowship Travel Program was created for full-time academic clinical faculty from foreign countries, providing them an opportunity to meet with St. Jude staff, observe them at work and learn about the hospital facility. Each year, five to six faculty members from other countries use the program.

Even before St. Jude Children's Research Hospital opened, ALSAC created an endowment of $300,000 for a chair at the University of Tennessee Memphis (UTM), the state's primary medical school, for the director of St. Jude.

Through the years, the university and hospital's collaboration has had varying degrees of success, resulting in a renewed commitment today to make that bond closer than ever. Many St. Jude faculty members (full-time staff M.D.s or Ph.D.s) hold faculty status in the graduate programs at UTM, and joint programs with the university provide UTM graduate students access to specialized research laboratories and techniques at St. Jude as part of their thesis work in molecular and cell biology, enzymology, virology and immunology. Moreover residents from UTM come to St. Jude to receive training in diagnostic imaging, hematology-oncology, infectious diseases, pathology, radiation oncology and surgery.

St. Jude's educational opportunities even extend to the high school level. Since 1982, an NIH grant has supported the Minority High School Student Apprentice Program. Each summer the program allows students, accompanied by their teachers, to gain first-hand experience in a health care and research environment.

Teaching takes many forms at St. Jude Children's Research Hospital. In addition to offering an opportunity for recently graduated doctors and scientists to continue their training at the hospital and pairing undergraduate students at the University of Tennessee Memphis with St. Jude faculty, St. Jude doctors and scientists take their knowledge on the road, traveling throughout the United States and world at large. Even when international diplomatic relations were strained, St. Jude faculty members have actively exchanged information with scientists around the globe. As early as 1972, Dr. Allan Granoff was telling the story of St. Jude to scientists in what was then the USSR. And in 1979, scientists from the Soviet Union came to Memphis to study influenza viruses at the hospital.

That same year, Dr. Alvin Mauer was invited to serve on an advisory board for cancer research for the King Faisal Specialist Hospital and Research Center in Saudi Arabia. Dr. Mauer also traveled to Libya as a participant in an international seminar commemorating UNICEF's International Year of the Child.

In 1972, Dr. Robert Webster, director of influenza studies at St. Jude, traveled to the People's Republic of China to address the Chinese Medical Academy in Beijing and assist Chinese scientists in establishing epidemiological studies of influenza viruses. This visit, the first of several by St. Jude doctors, initiated a research collaboration that included reciprocal laboratory visits and plans for training postdoctoral investigators. In 1980, Dr. Mauer visited China as a guest of the Chinese Academy of Medical Sciences. As a result of that visit, St. Jude and the academy established three special fellowships for postdoctoral trainees from China — in biochemistry, immunology and virology.

More recently, Dr. Malcolm Brenner, director of the bone marrow trans-

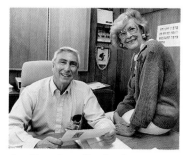

Dr. Allan Granoff and Helen Hogan, March 9, 1987. Both were among the first on the staff of St. Jude. Dr. Granoff was one of the first scientists recruited by Dr. Pinkel. Helen Hogan began as a volunteer with the Ladies of St. Jude, and shortly after the hospital opened she became a full time secretary.

plant program at St. Jude, was invited to Tokyo to meet with the Japanese Ministry of Health in the summer of 1993. Brenner was asked to advise the Japanese on gene therapy, an area of cancer research that they were preparing to enter.

The hospital's many years of participation in international meetings, its teaching visits to foreign nations, its on-site visits from foreign doctors and scientists, and its training of outstanding foreign doctors and scientists have given St. Jude an international reputation for excellence. Throughout the years, ALSAC has cited the hospital's international outreach as part of its appeal. So when a formally titled international outreach program was established in 1995, it took the goal of spreading information around the globe a step further. By sending St. Jude physicians of similar ethnicity to foreign countries where they can help structure patient care according to St. Jude protocols, hospital faculty are actively participating in the care of patients far from their Memphis clinics. Through this program, the hospital hopes to achieve cure rates abroad that are relatively comparable to those achieved at the Memphis facility. In this way, many more sick children will be touched by the caring hands of St. Jude.

The hospital's first outreach program, begun at St. Jude in the 1960s, focused not on communities abroad, but rather on the local Memphis population. At that time, Memphis was a city plagued by one of the highest infant mortality rates in the nation. During the crisis days of 1968, after Dr. Martin Luther King Jr. was assassinated in the city, members of the St. Jude staff felt it was their duty to address some of the problems immediately outside the hospital's doors. With this in mind they set up a clinic for children from Memphis' poorer communities, seeing them after-hours on their own time. After the clinic was established, it became clear that one of the major problems facing the city's poor was malnutrition. To address the situation, the St. Jude physicians teamed up with MAP-South (Memphis Area Project-South, a community organization aimed at breaking the poverty cycle) to provide food and medical care to the community.

In addition, Dr. Paul Zee, chief of nutrition at St. Jude, who had personally experienced hunger in Europe during WWII, began greatly accelerating his studies on the effects of malnutrition in children. For Dr. Pinkel and the Board of Governors, malnutrition constituted a catastrophic illness and should be deemed a part of the hospital's research program. To the St. Jude researchers, malnutrition was unconstitutional, unethical and immoral.

The St. Jude studies showed that a child's mental and physical growth pattern was established in the first six months of life. As a result of these findings, an infant formula was developed that was provided free to needy parents of children born at the City of Memphis Hospital.

To address malnutrition in older children, a supplemental food program was set up by MAP-South, and children who were enrolled in the program participated in studies conducted by the St. Jude research teams. The patients were examined at the general pediatric clinic at St. Jude and then followed through staff visits to their homes. In cases of severe malnutrition, patients were hospitalized. "We fed them and gave them a lot of TLC," says Lennie Lott, a pediatric nurse practitioner who assisted Dr. Zee and the other St. Jude doctors involved in the MAP-South Supplemental Feeding Program. Lott describes the children as having small heads, since their skulls had pre-

Dr. Cliona Rooney, seated, and Dr. Helen Heslop check diagnostic imaging results.

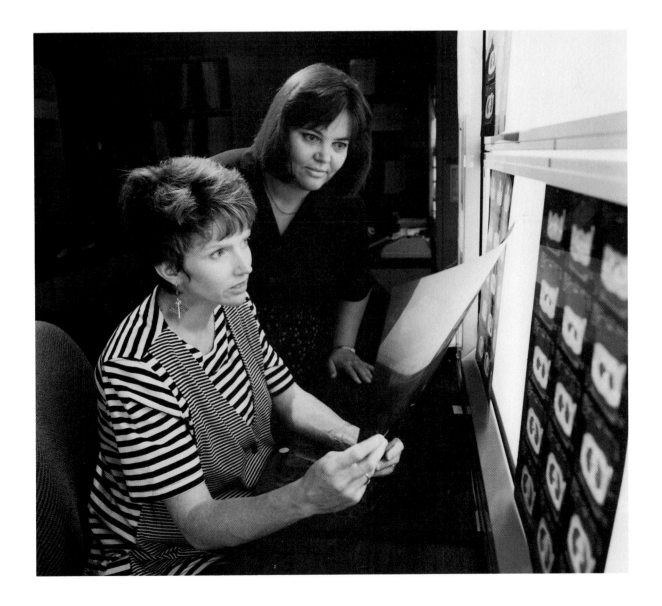

maturely molded due to inadequate nutrition. Yet serial skull X-rays taken during their treatment showed that their sutures were opening. "That was really wonderful to have been able to influence that child's growth and development at that point," Lott explains.

By demonstrating for the first time the effectiveness of supplemental feeding programs for improving the health of children at risk, the program sparked a great deal of interest around the community, resulting in a documentary filmed by Memphis television station WMC-TV. This documentary was seen in national syndication by Senator Hubert Humphrey of Minnesota. Humphrey's interest in the program led to legislation, supported by St. Jude data, that resulted in the establishment of the WIC (Women, Infant and Child) Supplemental Feeding Program, which has provided food for millions of needy people across the nation ever since. Through its ground-breaking studies, St. Jude Children's Research Hospital had made a difference in the lives of not just childhood cancer victims, but children suffering from hunger all over the United States.

Lott has watched the effects of the program in the Memphis area over the years, seeing many of its benefits extend beyond a child's physical improvements. Some of the program's patients have been able to move away from the ghetto and attend prestigious universities. "It made a change in quite a few of our children's lives, and their mothers' — their families' — lives," she notes. "And if you see a change in one or two, I think it's worth the effort."

Whether through a symposium aimed at acquainting referring physicians with the hospital's latest treatment protocols, a fellowship program for postdoctoral study, or a staff visit to El Salvador to help doctors there increase survival rates for ALL, St. Jude continues to share important information about its methods and research findings with doctors, nurses and scientists around the world. Through its research, education and outreach, St. Jude's mission has extended well beyond the walls of its clinics and laboratories, impacting children both across the street and countries away from its Memphis address.

Here are a few high points in the history of research at St. Jude:

• St. Jude's Total Therapy V Pilot Study was one of the most important contributions ever made in the treatment of childhood leukemia. Instituted in the early 1960s, the therapy eventually became a standard by which other studies around the world were measured. This study incorporated the best available elements from irradiation and chemotherapy in an aggressive, comprehensive approach. For the first time ever, half of the children treated for acute lymphoblastic leukemia (ALL) were alive and without evidence of disease

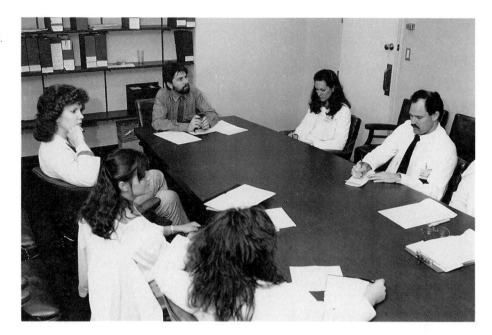

Typical staff conference of the leukemia service, 1987.

five years later. This study firmly established the three-phase approach to ALL therapy still used today: remission induction, central nervous system prophylaxis and continuation therapy.

• The first immunologic method to diagnose solid tumors in children was developed in 1965 at St. Jude by Dr. Warren Johnson.

• In 1968, St. Jude researchers led by Dr. Omar Hustu found chemotherapy was effective against Ewing sarcoma, one of the most frequent malignant bone tumors in children. Chemotherapy was then combined with radiation, which led to a significant improvement in the survival rate of Ewing sarcoma patients.

• In 1975, St. Jude became the first hospital to recognize that not all children with ALL had the same type of disease. Researchers, led by Dr. Louis Borella, identified important subtypes of ALL, an observation that led to studies around the world designed to provide biological explanations for clinical observations that the disease followed many different patterns in identically treated patients. This finding that ALL was not a single disease led to better classifications into standard-risk and high-risk ALL, resulting in new research directions and improved treatment.

• In 1975, Dr. Gaston Rivera and his research team discovered a new drug combination that would attack leukemia that had recurred after initial treatment. This led to improved therapy for thousands of leukemia patients, especially those with a very high risk of early failure.

• The second most common solid tumor in children, neuroblastoma, was tackled by St. Jude researchers in the 1970s. In 1977, investigators developed a treatment effective for more than half of patients with this type of solid tumor.

• Once researchers identified cancer therapies that were potentially cures, they faced another monumental challenge. Because cancer treatments lower the body's immune response, drugs that offered the only hope of survival were at the same time subjecting children to the threat of death from infection. One of these infections was a pneumonia caused by the then little-known organism *Pneumocystis carinii*, which could be fatal to a child receiving chemotherapy. In 1977, Dr. Walter Hughes and his research group developed a treatment, using the drug TMP-SMZ, that not only stopped *Pneumocystis carinii* pneumonia, but could also prevent it and other bacterial infections from occurring. The treatment was hailed nationally as a great success and became a standard preventive measure for a variety of patients at risk for this lethal infection. The treatment has been almost 100 percent effective. The victory over *P. carinii* is considered one of the hospital's true medical breakthroughs and has saved thousands of patients who were cured of cancer but at high risk for this usually fatal pneumonia. And since *P. carinii* pneumonia is one of the leading diseases of AIDS patients, Dr. Hughes' team became one of the earliest to investigate new drugs for use with infections in cases of pediatric AIDS.

• In 1984, under Dr. Thomas Look, St. Jude faculty members discovered a novel method to identify patients with neuroblastoma who are likely to have a poor response to therapy. This discovery allows therapists to concentrate on this high-risk group while sparing lower-risk patients from the toxicity associated with intensive treatment.

Dr. Pam Hinds leads nursing conference in April 1988. With her Ph.D. in nursing, Dr. Hinds heads St. Jude's nursing research programs.

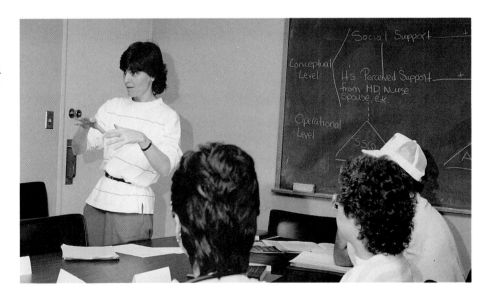

• Another discovery about the way certain patients respond to cancer treatment was found in 1984, when Dr. Dorothy Williams learned that a rearrangement of the genetic material within human chromosomes is an important factor in how a child with leukemia responds to treatment.

• Evidence of the existence of a "hybrid" leukemia, a mixture of acute myeloid and acute lymphoblastic leukemia, was discovered in 1984 at St. Jude by Dr. Joseph Mirro.

• Children who are able to retain drugs longer in higher concentrations are more likely to become long-term survivors. This evidence that the curability of childhood leukemia depends on the availability of anticancer drugs within the body once they have been administered was discovered at St. Jude by Dr. William Evans in 1984.

• In 1985, Dr. Charles Sherr found alterations in the gene that codes for a growth factor receptor of certain types of white blood cells. This was pivotal because these alterations provide the basis for the transformation of normal cells into leukemia cells and for their subsequent spread throughout the body.

• A new anticancer drug, 2-Chlorodeoxyadenosine (2-CDA), was found effective in pediatric patients with relapsed acute myeloid leukemia (AML) in 1988 by Drs. Raymond Blakley and Victor Santana. This discovery was enormously important in the treatment of AML, a generally drug-resistant disease in children and adults.

• Another advance in the treatment of AML was discovered at St. Jude in 1990. Dr. Ching-Hon Pui found that risk of development of secondary AML, a then-emerging problem in children initially treated for ALL, was found to be low or negligible in children treated for malignant solid tumors.

• Radioactive implants were first used successfully to treat childhood brain tumors in 1990 by a St. Jude research team led by Drs. James Fontanesi and Larry Kun.

• The discovery of blood cell growth factors, known as CSFs, or colony stimulating factors, in 1990 at St. Jude will play an important role in the future management of childhood solid tumors. These CSFs were found to counteract life-threatening bone marrow depletion caused by the toxic effects of intensive chemotherapy.

• In 1990, St. Jude researchers also found the first evidence that an antimalarial drug can prevent or effectively treat a life-threatening form of pneumonia in AIDS patients.

• In 1991, the overall long-term survival rates of ALL patients were shown to have increased from 50 percent to 73 percent, thanks to a new treatment approach. This involved intensive induction therapy followed by more than two years of treatment with eight anticancer drugs. Dr. Gaston Rivera and his team of investigators also noted advances in several of the toughest-to-cure groups: babies, adolescents and children of African-American descent.

• Dr. Laura Bowman found in a 1991 survey that neuroblastoma treatment at St. Jude over the previous 25 years had led to a 25 percent improvement in the survival rates for children with this solid tumor. The survival rate now reaches 57 percent.

• An improved dosage regimen which virtually eliminates the risk of secondary AML in patients treated with the drugs known as VM26 and VP16 was developed at St. Jude in 1991.

• A sometimes-deadly side effect of chemotherapy is a severe decrease in white blood cells. In 1991, St. Jude researchers discovered that a blood stimulating agent, known as GM-CSF, can help children escape this side effect. Doctors hope the compound may also save lives by allowing them to give higher doses of powerful anticancer drugs. Studies have shown that patients who have been given high doses of GM-CSF need fewer days of antibiotic treatment and are less likely than those receiving lower doses to be hospitalized for fever after chemotherapy.

• In 1992, St. Jude announced a cooperative effort to form a pediatric AIDS Clinical Trials Unit with two other Memphis area hospitals. The ACTU provides access to drug trials for the growing number of HIV-infected children in the nation's middle and Southern states.

• Dr. Mary Ellen Conley identified key genes in 1992 involved in two immunodeficiency diseases in male children. This was a major contribution to the knowledge of hereditary disorders. Collaborative studies provided precise diagnostic probes for use in genetic counseling and provided information useful to the long-term possibility of gene therapy.

• In 1992, St. Jude virologists Maria Castrucci and Yoshihiro Kawaoka showed that the genetic makeup of a live influenza virus can be changed in a way that makes it much less virulent. Live virus vaccines provide superior protection, but can also produce symptoms or even full-blown influenza. The ability to manipulate key viral genes opens the way for the development of a safe, effective live vaccine. Ultimately, it should be possible to design a live vaccine that combines the desirable elements of natural infection without any of its hazards.

• The World Health Organization first established its animal flu virus identification center at St. Jude in 1975. Under the direction of Dr. Robert

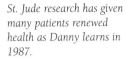

St. Jude research has given many patients renewed health as Danny learns in 1987.

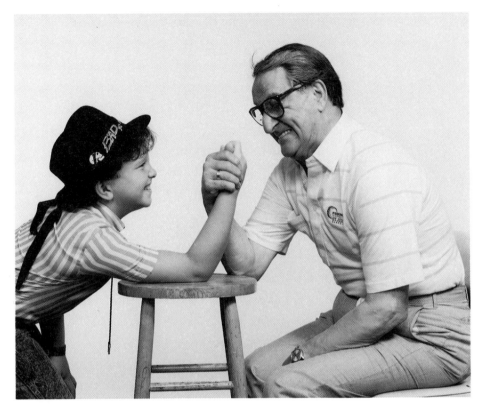

Webster, St. Jude researchers collaborated with WHO in a study that identified wild aquatic fowl as the source of genes for the influenza viruses that infect other species, including humans.

• In 1992, St. Jude Children's Research Hospital became the first center outside the National Institutes of Health approved to use gene transfer technology in a clinical trial. Dr. Malcolm Brenner and colleagues genetically marked cells to determine the source of relapses that occur after high-dose chemotherapy and bone marrow rescue via autologous transplantation. Results showed that undetected malignant cells in the transplanted marrow, harvested during clinical remission, are responsible for some relapses. In 1994, Dr. Brenner and his colleagues received regulatory approval to study a gene-transfer-based therapy in children with advanced neuroblastoma. The "tumor vaccine" created by this technology has shown promising activity in these preliminary studies.

• HIV infections were first shown to be preventable by chemotherapy at St. Jude in 1994. The AIDS Clinical Trials Unit participated in a study that showed, for the first time, that infants are at a lower risk of acquiring HIV when a drug called ziduvodine, or AZT, is given to infected women during pregnancy and to newborns. The trial was so successful that it was stopped early so that all participants and others in similar situations could have the benefits of the study's discovery at the earliest possible date.

• Targeted T-cells — T-cells engineered to seek out and fight a specific problem — were first used as a cell therapy against Epstein-Barr virus lymphoma in 1994. Although the bone marrow transplant process has improved drastically, patients receiving transplants are vulnerable to a range of infections during the immediate post-transplant period. EBV-specific T-cells are developed and administered to patients who have received T-cell depleted transplants to fight EBV infections and its resultant lymphoma, a cancer of the lymphatic system's lymphoid tissue, without inducing graft-versus-host disease. This treatment can reverse the life-threatening lymphoma, and prevent its development in patients at risk.

• In 1995, survival rates for African-American children were shown to have reached parity with Caucasian children when treated with a therapy based on a St. Jude protocol. This improvement is mostly based on advances made in the survival rates for African-American children treated for acute lymphocytic leukemia.

• Some cancer patients are deficient in a substance known as TPMT, which makes them unable to metabolize a common chemotherapy drug known as mercaptopurine. In 1995, researchers were able to identify the genetic defect responsible for TPMT deficiency. Now, patients who might have received toxic amounts of mercaptopurine before their sensitivity to it was discovered can learn of their TPMT deficiency through a DNA assay devised at St. Jude.

An Album of
Hope

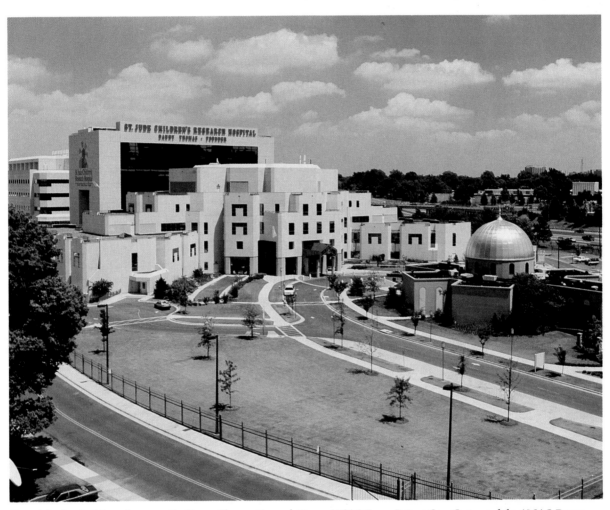

From left edge, buildings shown are the Danny Thomas Research Tower, ALSAC Tower, Patient Care Center and the ALSAC-Danny Thomas Pavilion.

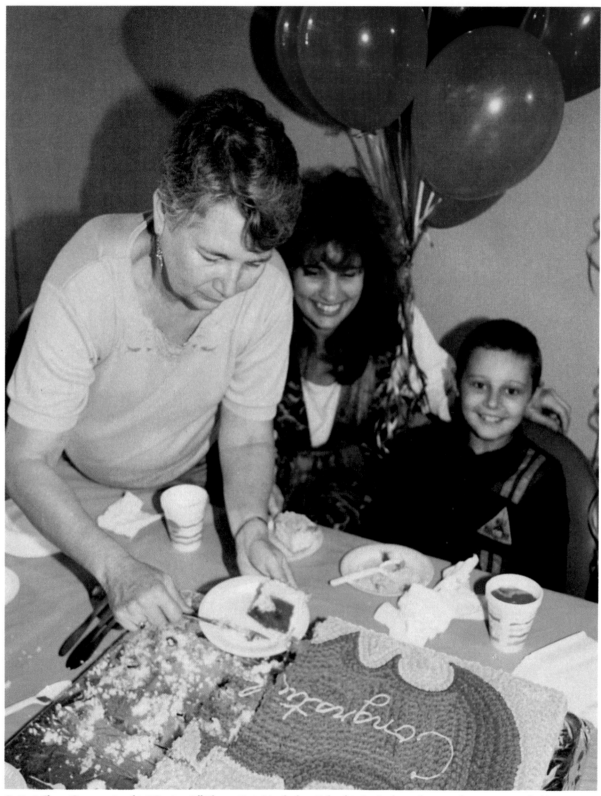

Patient Chase George enjoys his "Coming Off Chemo Party" in the hospital cafeteria. In the early years there was no such thing as "coming off chemotherapy" — being taken off all anti-cancer drugs — but thanks to its research St. Jude now gives many of these parties.

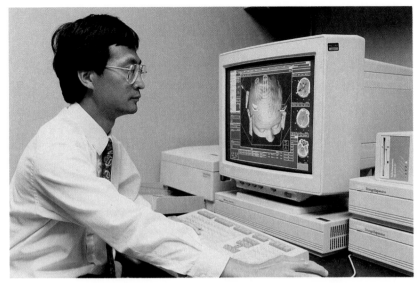

Diagnostic imaging relies heavily on computer generated views.

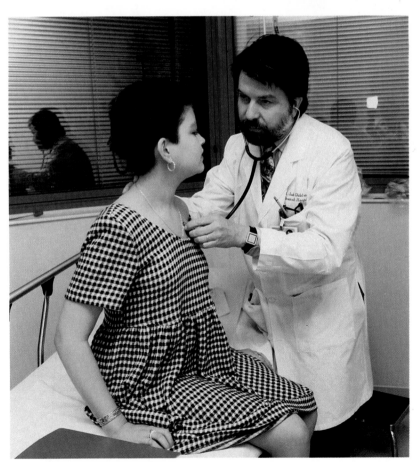

Dr. Gaston Rivera examines Tady Cruz, 1994.

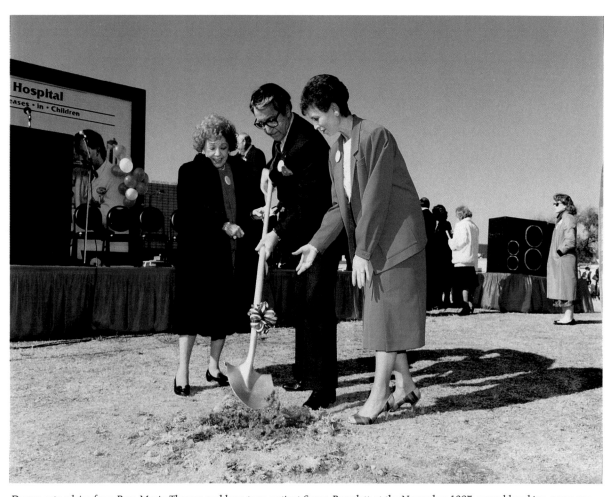

Danny gets advice from Rose Marie Thomas and long-term patient Susan Bramlett at the November 1987 ground breaking ceremony for the start of the hospital s multi-million dollar expansion program.

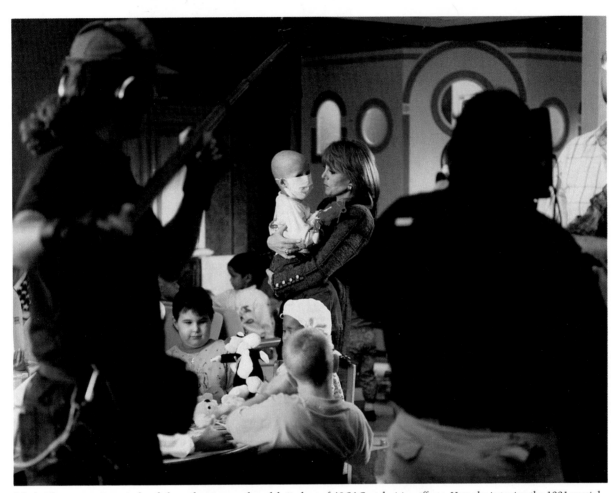

Marlo Thomas continues in her father's footsteps as the celebrity host of ALSAC's television efforts. Here she is taping the 1991 special in the waiting area that was temporarily housed on the ground floor of the Danny Thomas Research Tower while the new patient care center was being built. Her co-host, actor John Goodman, donated his service for this very productive hour-long show.

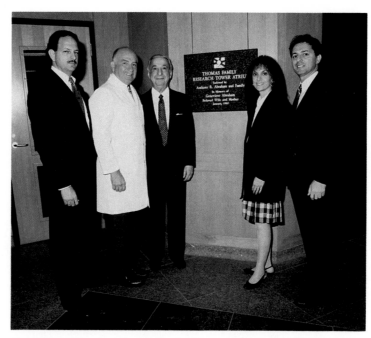

Terre Thomas represents the Thomas family at one of the many dedications in the new buildings at St. Jude. From left, Bill Maloof, Dr. Simone, Anthony Abraham, Terre and Tom Abraham dedicate the atrium of the research tower in memory of Genevieve Abraham in 1992.

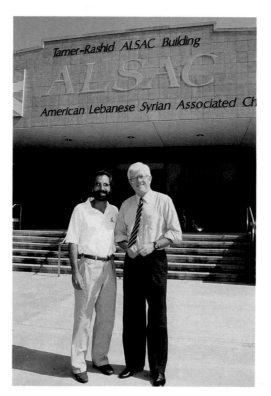

Tony Thomas and Phil Donahue, husband of Marlo Thomas, are regular participants in celebrity events for St. Jude. Here they pose in front of ALSAC headquarters before playing in the pro-am round of the 1993 FedEx St. Jude Classic.

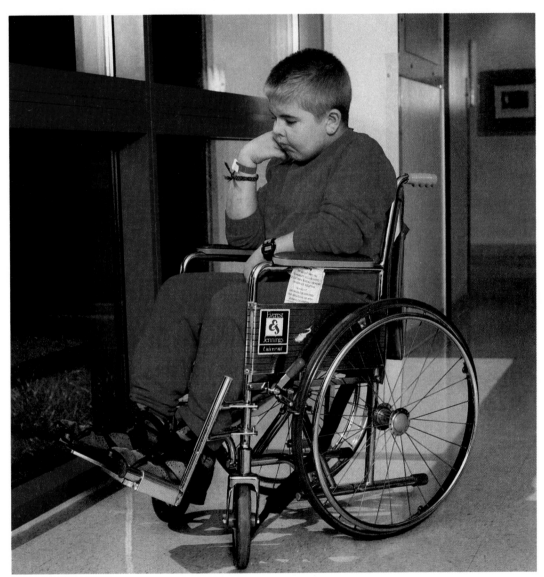

Patient thoughts are not always meant to be shared.

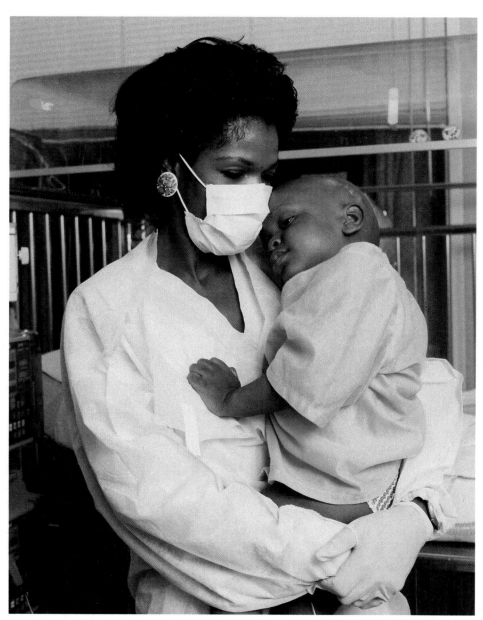

Linda Jones comforts Larry Sutton.

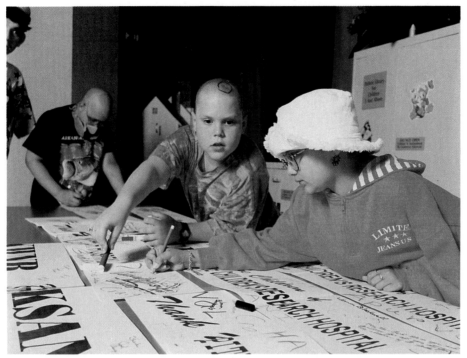

Patients frequently show their appreciation by signing banners and greetings to be used in various ALSAC events.

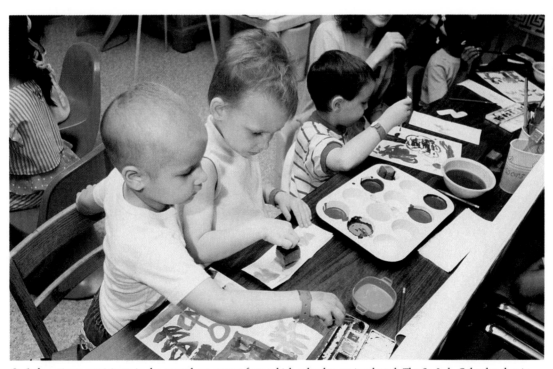

St. Jude patients participate in the annual art contest from which calendar art is selected. The St. Jude Calendar that is sent to major donors as a "thank you" for their support. Recipients are never asked for a donation in the calendar mailing, but from its start in 1985, the calendar, produced by ALSAC's communications department, has generated four to five times its total cost in unsolicited gifts.

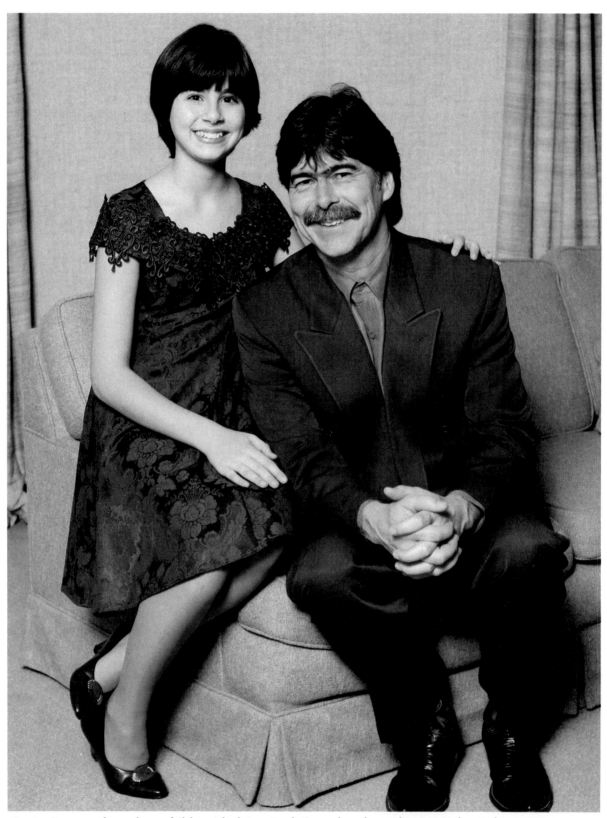

Country Cares came from a dream of Alabama's lead singer Randy Owen, shown here with patient Lindsey Cook.

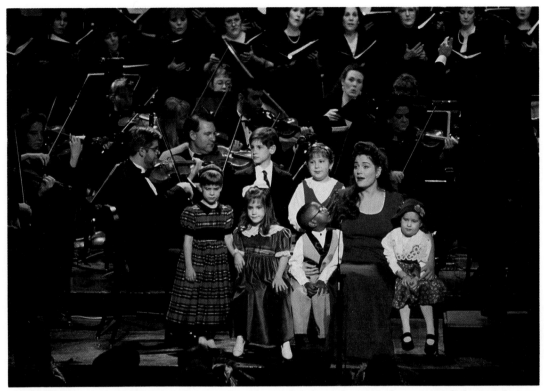

Patients join opera star Kallen Esperian on stage for "Silent Night" during her 1995 Christmas benefit for St. Jude.

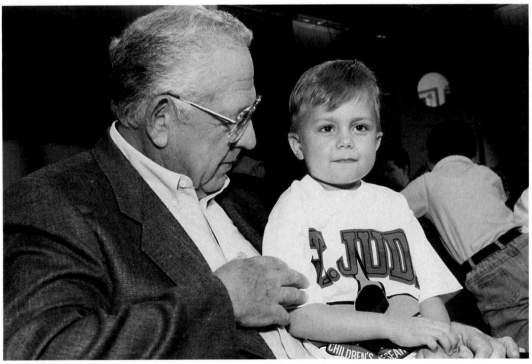

St. Jude board member R. David Thomas visits with patient in April 1995.

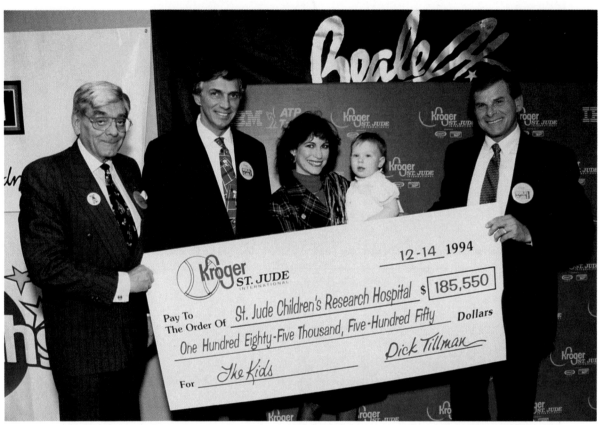

Fund raising activities such as the Kroger St. Jude tennis tournament bring in thousands of dollars each year to aid the hospital's efforts.

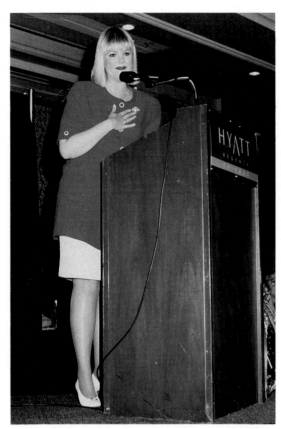

Actress Ann Jillian, a supporter of St. Jude, speaks to the delegates at 1991 convention.

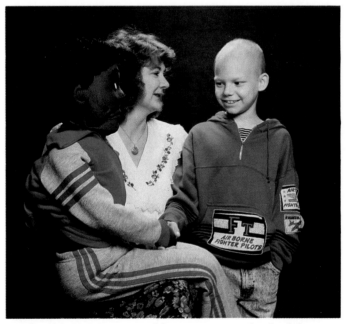

Social worker Fran Greeson uses life-size puppet named Will to help patient Robert Dupree.

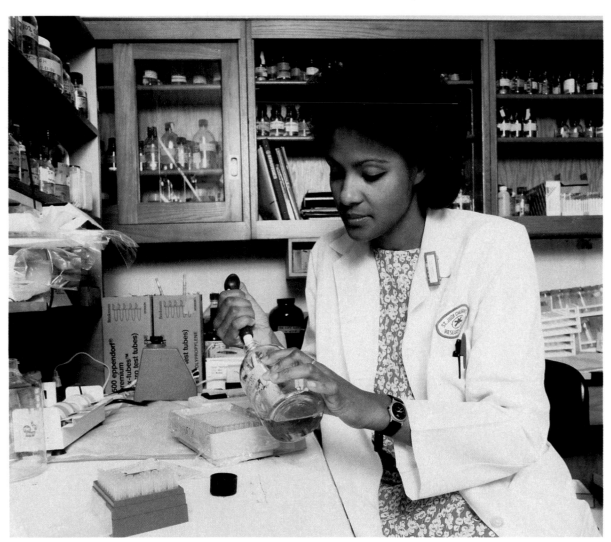

Ruth Ann Scroggs in virology lab.

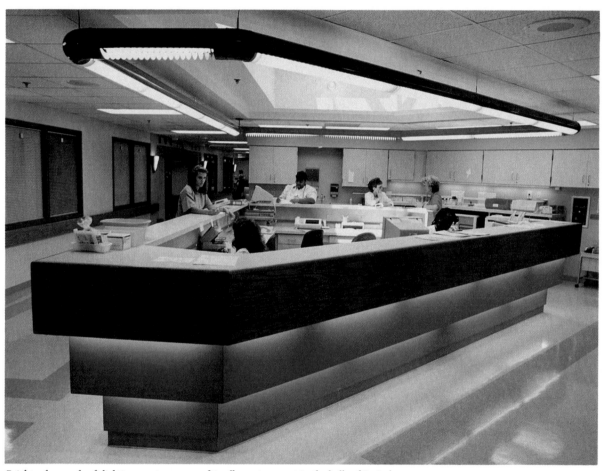

Bright colors and soft lighting create a warm, friendly environment in the halls of St. Jude.

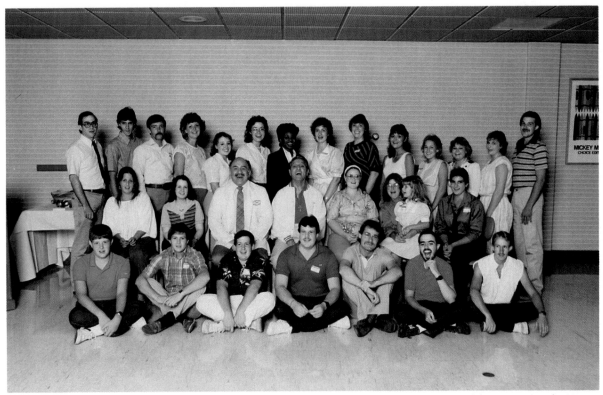

First "alumni" reunion, June 1985. Long term survivors meet in original cafeteria with Danny Thomas and director Dr. Joseph V. Simone.

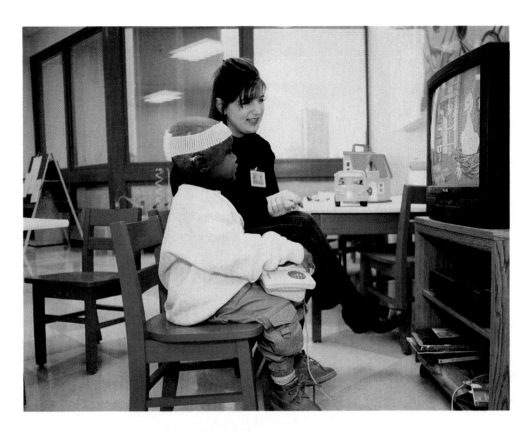

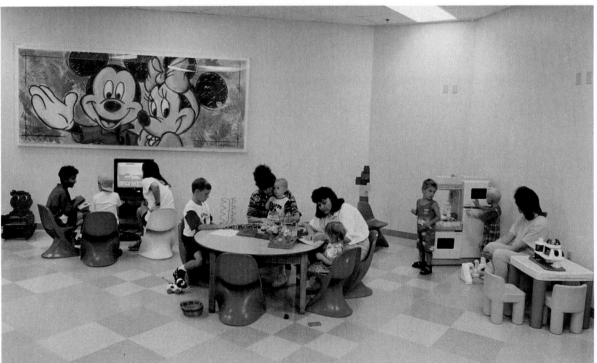

Bright, well-equipped recreation rooms provide distraction as well as therapy for children in treatment. Staff, volunteers, friends and family all join in.

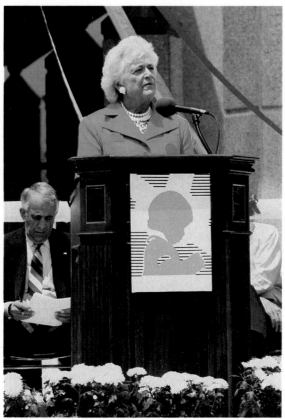

Barbara Bush delivers the keynote address at the dedication of the Danny Thomas Research Tower, 1991.

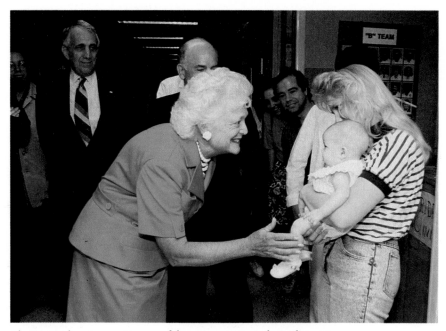

The First Lady enjoys meeting one of the younger patients during her visit.

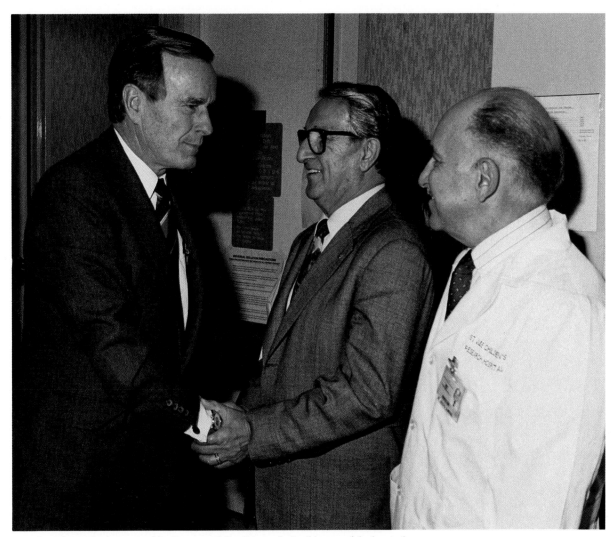

President George Bush is greeted by Danny and Dr. Simone during his tour of the hospital.

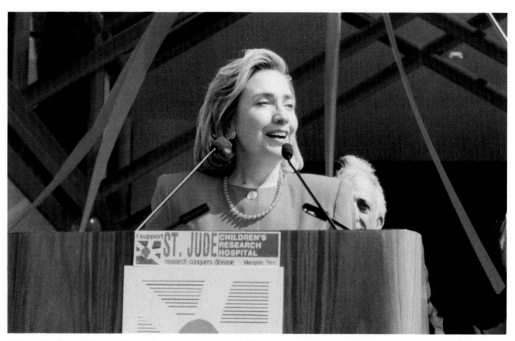

Hillary Rodham Clinton delivers keynote address at dedication of new patient care center, October 1994.

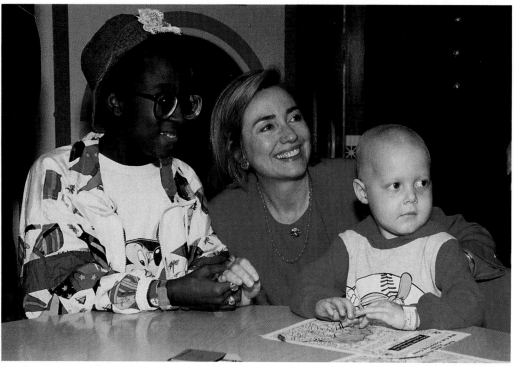

Another First Lady offering cheer and support to patients.

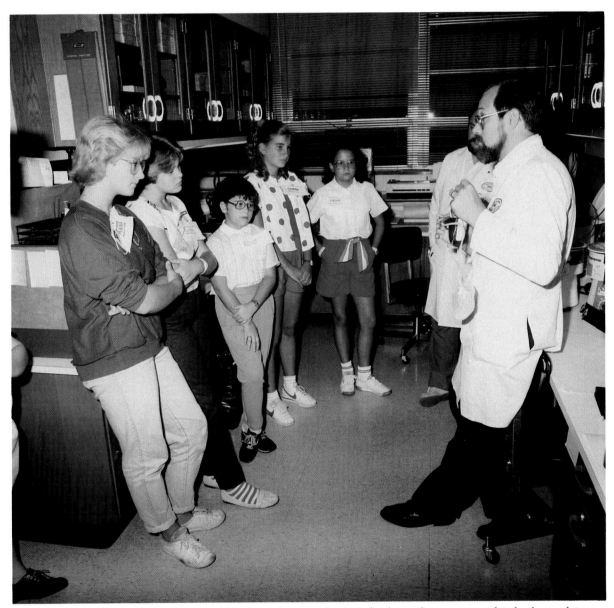

Keith Kunkel briefs patient siblings during St. Jude Sibs Week. During this event they learn what to expect as their brothers and sisters receive treatment, and what they can do to help.

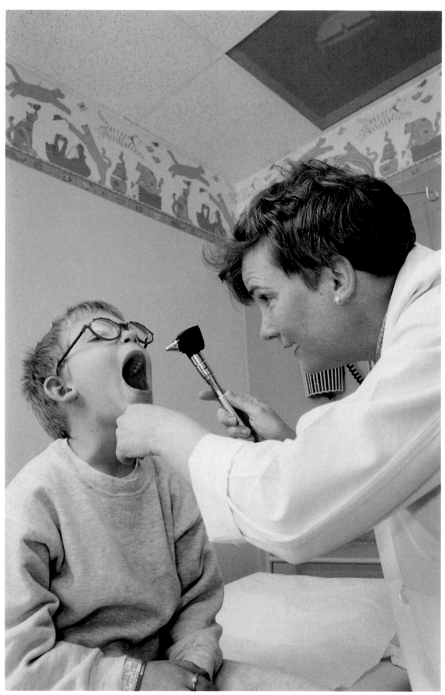

Chemotherapy may affect parts of the patient's body other than the target area. Dental care is especially important, and it is among the support treatments provided.

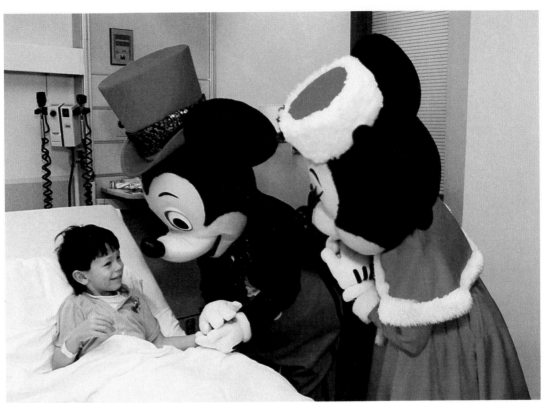

Patients are often treated to visits by celebrities dear to their hearts. These have included Muhammad Ali, Michael Jackson, Bugs Bunny and, of course, Mickey and Minnie Mouse.

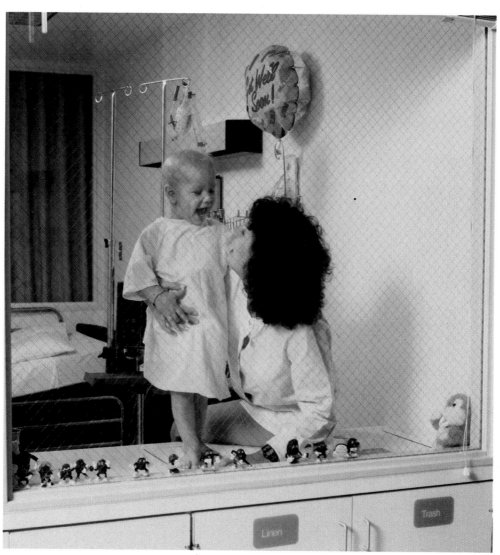

Nurse Vanessa Howard with Cody Burks

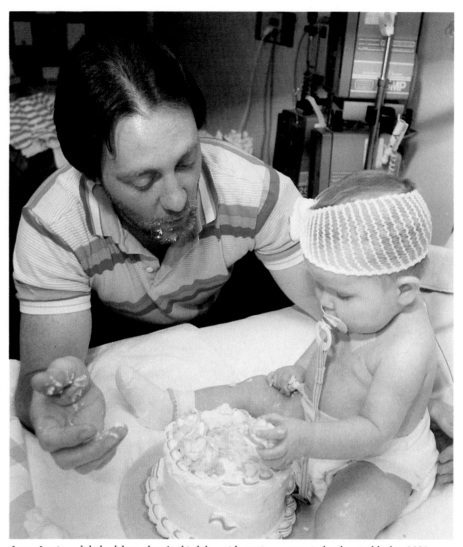

Jenna Lewis and dad celebrate her 1st birthday with a private party in her hospital bed in 1991.

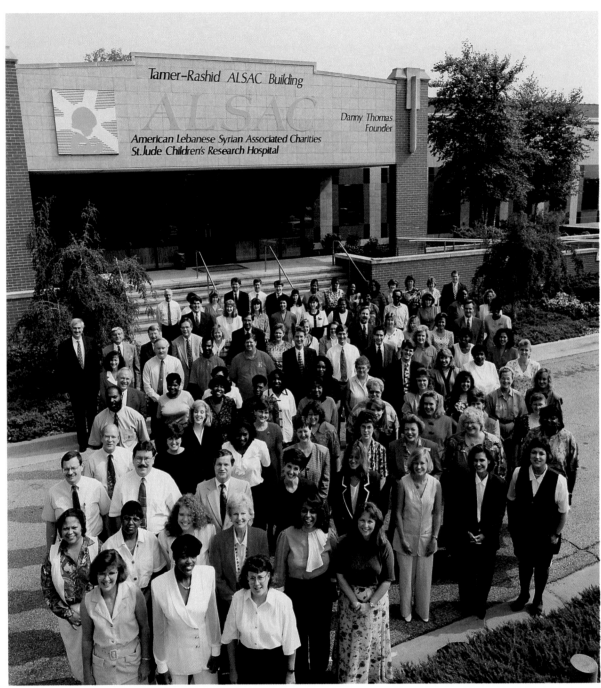

With fewer than 200 full-time employees nationwide, ALSAC has one of the highest dollars raised per employee ratios of any national charity. This 1996 photo in front of the Memphis headquarters shows the majority of ALSAC's staff.

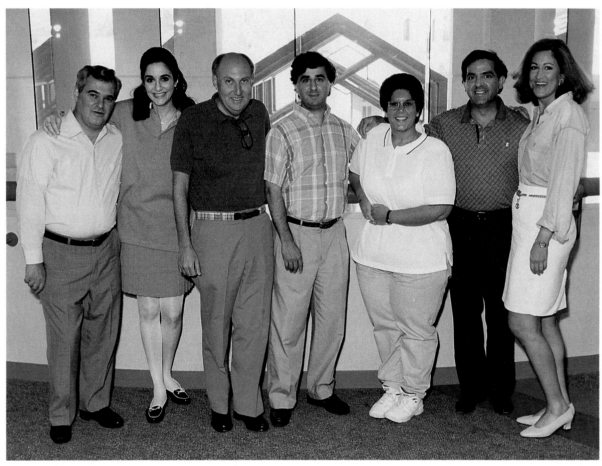

Sons and daughters of original ALSAC-St. Jude board members are now earning places on the national board. From left, Paul Hajar, Dr. Susan Aguillard, Fred P. Gattas, Jr., Anthony Shaker, Joyce Aboussie, Joseph G. Shaker, and Judy Habib are among those children of founders now serving. Also serving but not pictured are Joseph Ayoub, Jr., Paul Ayoub, John Bourisk, Jr., Fred Harris, Rochelle Joseph, George Simon II, Paul Simon, and Terre Thomas.

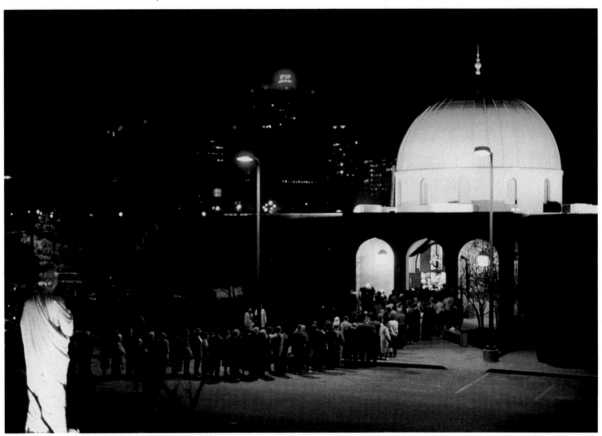

Thousands stood in line for hours in bitter cold to pay their respects to Danny at the pavilion on Feb. 9, 1991. Memphis police estimated that the lines stretched for more than one mile.

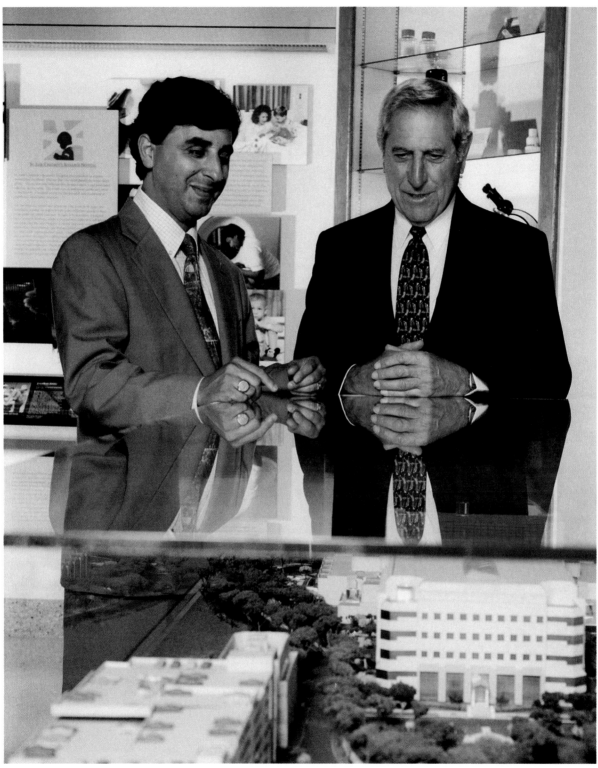

Board members Anthony Shaker, left, and Joe Haggar discuss model of the hospital's expansion plan during 1994 board meeting in Memphis.

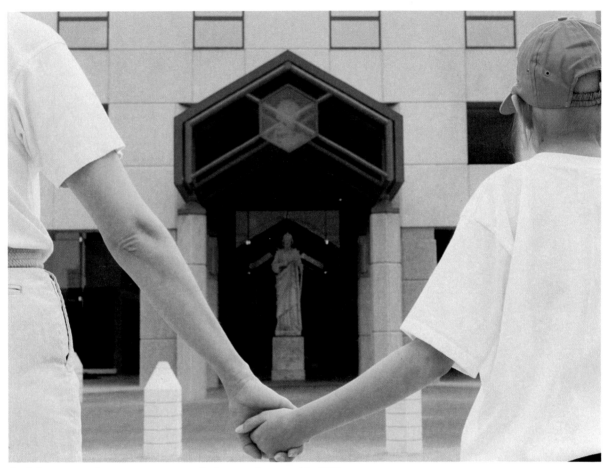

St. Jude statue stands at entrance to new patient care center opened in 1995.

BRICKS AND MORTAR, CONCRETE AND STEEL

We thought the hospital would cost $2,500,000 — when the research wing is completed this fall, it will have cost $6,000,000. We expected the maintenance to be $500,000 a year — by October it will cost us $100,000 a month to keep St. Jude in operation.
— **Michael F. Tamer letter, May 21, 1962**

On the north side of Interstate 40 in downtown Memphis, immediately before the expressway traverses the Hernando De Soto Bridge connecting Tennessee with Arkansas, stand a group of four large pink buildings and a smaller gold-domed pavilion. This is St. Jude Children's Research Hospital. The hospital's eye-catching structures are as much a landmark today as the original star-shaped hospital was in the early 1960s. St. Jude's facilities, like the life-saving work carried on behind its walls, reflect the innovative way of thinking that has characterized the hospital since its ground breaking on November 2, 1958.

The forethought used in planning the hospital went far beyond the realm of medicine and science. Engineers for the original structure recognized early on that Memphis was located on a major earthquake fault, with the potential for severe damage in the event of a temblor. It was thus decided that St. Jude would be built to resist Zone 3 earthquake damage, the first building in the city to follow the uniform building code. (In addition to making it one of the most earthquake-resistant buildings in the area, this had the unanticipated consequence of making its demolition take longer when it was razed in 1992.)

St. Jude was also the first completely desegregated hospital in the Memphis area. Black and white patients were treated in the same rooms; black and white parents waited together; dining and bathroom facilities were integrated; black doctors treated white patients. Cardinal Stritch had emphasized the importance of a desegregated facility open to all children, no matter what their race, when he and Danny first spoke of the hospital, and Danny insisted that St. Jude be a non-sectarian, desegregated facility. The idea was grounded in

Thomas' belief that all children, no matter what their background, should be given a fighting chance. Bud Rashid, ALSAC's national executive director from 1976 to 1992, says, "I think that Danny saw the poverty in the Midsouth area, he saw the amount of sickle cell anemia among black children in that area, and he saw the amount of illness, particularly leukemia, among the poor people in the South, and he just was determined he was going to get that medical aid available to them."

The open-door policy was instituted and upheld from the time the hospital began operations. Even though there was still discrimination in the South, it was not going to be permitted at St. Jude. "We felt like this was a nationwide institution, given to the United States by people of Middle Eastern background," comments Rashid, "and therefore we wanted it to be available to all people in the United States."

From its beginnings, the hospital truly reflected the grace of its patron saint. For Danny Thomas, even the original design itself was yet be another example of St. Jude's intervention. Noted black architect Paul Williams of Los Angeles but born in Memphis claimed he had no idea that the five-pointed star was the symbol of St. Jude when he drew and donated the plans. "Some people call this nice coincidence," said Danny at the time. "I call it the hand of God pushing Williams' pencil."

The building was designed with five wings radiating from a central hub. The hub was to house the outpatient department, staff offices, records room, blood bank, admitting offices, social services department and a small non-sectarian chapel. The second floor of the hub would contain administrative offices, housing for the resident staff and the sisters who were to administer the services of the hospital, assembly rooms for meetings, a medical library and schoolrooms for children who were patients.

Inpatient rooms accommodating 38 children; kitchen, dining room and related facilities; X-ray and clinical laboratories; surgical facilities and central supply units; and research offices and facilities were each to be housed in a separate wing. The basement was slated for research areas, shops, laundry, maintenance and a communications center that would include photography and art. Research space was left open so that it could be designed and utilized as the need arose.

In arranging the research facilities, Dr. Donald Pinkel, the hospital's first medical director, made one major change to the original plans. He eliminated the proposed surgical wing. Instead he made arrangements with next door neighbor St. Joseph Hospital to use its facilities for surgery, and a tunnel was built to

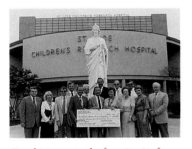

For thirty years, the favorite site for group pictures was in front of the statue of St. Jude Thaddeus. Thousands of checks from fund raising events like that of the Tennessee Telephone Pioneers in June 1985, were presented, and even more individual pictures were taken there.

In addition to their primary function of providing medical photographic support, the BioMedical Communications staff provides ALSAC with shots of the volunteer's check presentations. In 1987, they had their own group picture made.

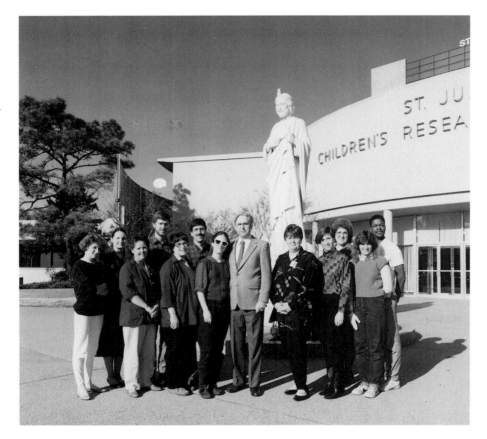

connect the two buildings. The wing designed for surgery would be utilized for research. That meant three of the five wings were devoted to laboratories, providing a maximum opportunity to bring clinical studies to the laboratory and laboratory studies to the Children's problems.

After the opening, the hospital's early medical success brought problems. Even with its sophisticated facilities, it was apparent by 1970 that St. Jude was running out of space. An ever-increasing patient roster, growing staff and increasing need for more research areas spurred plans for a $4 million, seven-story tower, announced in October 1971. By the time of the tower's completion in 1975, the actual cost had doubled to $8 million.

Three years after ground breaking in 1972, the new 118,000-square-foot tower was dedicated in November 1975. In addition to remarks by Danny Thomas, Ed Barry and other dignitaries, the ceremony included a taped message by President Gerald Ford, beginning a tradition of White House participation in St. Jude dedications. The building contained an auditorium, meeting rooms and two floors for in-patient care. The remainder of its much-needed space would be used for research. The inpatient wings of the original star-shaped building were converted to research facilities.

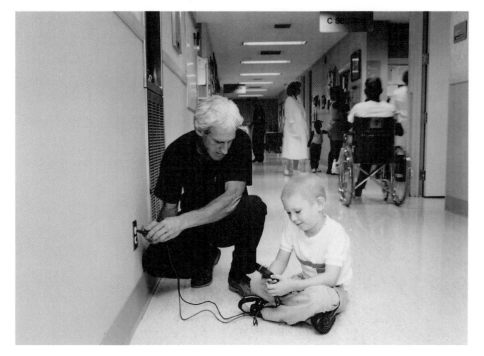

The early 1980s also brought more growth, starting with the completion
of America's most technologically sophisticated research building for handling
biological agents and laboratory research animals, dedicated on June 25, 1981.
Funds for this facility had been raised from the Memphis business community by
an ALSAC committee led by John Ford Canale. In his remarks at this dedication,
Danny Thomas said that St. Jude is a "harsh taskmaster. As soon as I get one thing
done, he tells me to do something else for this institution." Detroit industrialist
George Simon Sr., the chairman of the ALSAC Board that year, responded to
Danny's remark with, "Please, Danny, no more promises."

Even with the seven-story tower and the confinement facility, the hospital was again faced with the need for more space as its staff, patient and facilities
demands continued to grow. Materials and equiipment had to be stored in the
basement halls. Temporary buildings, some left from building contractors, were
used for engineering and biomedical communications, and mobile home offices
were placed on the grounds to house personnel and other administrative offices.
Space was constantly being filled, and new needs were constantly being created.
Moreover, the hospital's academic relationship with the University of Tennessee
Memphis had become less than adequate and was a source of frustration for the
St. Jude doctors and scientists. Thus as noted earlier, when the highly regarded
Washington University Medical Center invited St. Jude to relocate to St. Louis in
late 1984, it was viewed as a very attractive offer.

The discussions and board decisions generated by this invitation led to one of America's most extensive and unusual hospital construction programs, unusual in that it was done without the need for borrowing, and paid for as it was built. At its February 1986 meeting, the board accepted a committee report recommending that the expansion deemed necessary for continued advances by St. Jude be put in place on the Memphis site. This was the beginning of what was then estimated to be a $125,000,000 program designed to position St. Jude Children's Research Hospital to continue in its role as a medical and scientific leader into the 21st century. This turned out to be one of the largest hospital construction programs ever undertaken in America paid for on a pay-as-you-build basis, thanks to the dedication of ALSAC's professional staff and the millions of volunteers and donors all over America.

The hospital's goal to build a top-notch facility that would attract some of the world's leading doctors and scientists has paid off. In the last 10 years, St. Jude has recruited some extraordinarily strong scientists. Dr. Allan Granoff says, "I don't think there's any question about being able to hire the top people in the country (to come) here." Granoff says, "I think time has proved that we didn't need St. Louis (i.e. Washington University) to achieve whatever we wanted to achieve."

World-class scientists' arrival at St. Jude paves the way for additional recruits. "We now have very major figures in several fields at this institution," says Dr. Nienhuis. "And that helps a great deal [with recruitment]. It's because of the scientific atmosphere and because of the aid that ALSAC gives us."

With St. Jude's decision to remain in Memphis, Memphis businessman and ALSAC-St. Jude Board member Sam Cooper launched the 1986 Mission for Memphis fund-raising drive, making good on one of the promises the Memphis business community had given the board as an inducement to stay in Memphis. Cooper led the 1974 Mission For Memphis campaign that had raised money for the first expansion of the hospital. He enlisted Memphis real estate developer Jack Belz and Federal Express Chairman Fred Smith, both St. Jude board members, as co-chairmen in the $12.5 million 1986 drive. Ten million dollars of that money was earmarked for the expansion and renovation of the hospital, with $2.5 million designated to match funds from the State of Tennessee for the creation of new chairs of research excellence at the University of Tennessee Memphis Department of Pediatrics to complement the research at St. Jude. The 1986 Mission for Memphis ultimately raised $18.2 million from 250 local businesses.

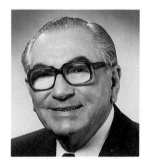

Sam Cooper (Photo courtesy Les & Ed Cooper Commercial Photographers)

The following year, on November 19, 1987, Danny Thomas, his wife, Rose Marie, and long time patient Susan Bramlett ceremonially broke ground for St. Jude Children's Research Hospital's expansion and renovation program as part

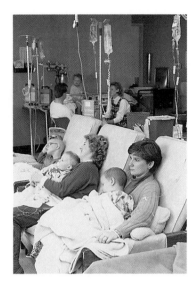

Children and their parents spend many hours receiving infusions at the hospital's medicine room. This is a typical day at the old medicine room in the 1980s.

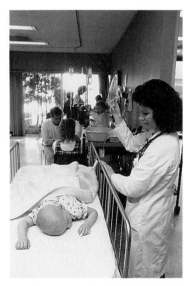

Another scene in the 1962 building's medicine room.

of the hospital's 25th and ALSAC's 30th anniversary observances. The expansion would more than double the hospital's size to 707,735 gross square feet, providing more research space and patient care rooms, as well as allowing for an increase in staff. The program included the demolition of the original hospital building and construction of a four-story Patient Care Center, five-story Danny Thomas Research Tower, central energy plant and 1,000-vehicle parking facility. The final phase of the project called for extensive renovations of the seven-story tower.

Today the hospital's expanded campus exhibits the result of what became a $155 million commitment. The 1,000-vehicle parking facility was completed in July 1989, and a one-story Magnetic Resonance Imaging (MRI) building, containing one of the most powerful magnets in North America, sits adjacent to the new Danny Thomas Research Tower. Here the hospital's diagnostic imaging staff conducts spectroscopy studies that provide new methods for evaluating patient responses to therapy.

The five-story Danny Thomas Research Tower was dedicated on June 14, 1991, an event attended by Danny's children — Marlo, Terre and Tony Thomas — and First Lady Barbara Bush, who gave the keynote speech.

With the opening of the research tower, a period of temporary moves akin to a large scale version of musical chairs began. The tower became the temporary, four-year home of the patient care clinics and administrative offices while the original hospital building was demolished and the new Patient Care Center was being built. Danny Thomas, who loved the original star-shaped building he called "the star of hope," fully approved of its sacrifice for the sake of improving care for the "children of St. Jude."

The Danny Thomas Research Tower now houses most of the basic science laboratories previously located in the 1975 research and inpatient care tower. These include St. Jude's departments of immunology, tumor cell biology, biochemistry, pharmacokinetics, virology/molecular biology and some divisions of hematology/oncology and pathology. The site also houses such support services as biomedical communications, biomedical engineering, electron microscopy, facilities management, ultra cold storage, radiation safety, the biomedical library and the copy center.

The hospital's basic science faculty worked closely with the building's architects in programming the tower for functionality and maximum use of space. Laboratory complexes surround a five-story atrium, allowing for optimum efficiency and flexibility. Every lab has its own ventilation system, and all walls in the labs are temporary for easy reconfiguration. With each floor con-

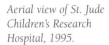

*Aerial view of St. Jude
Children's Research
Hospital, 1995.*

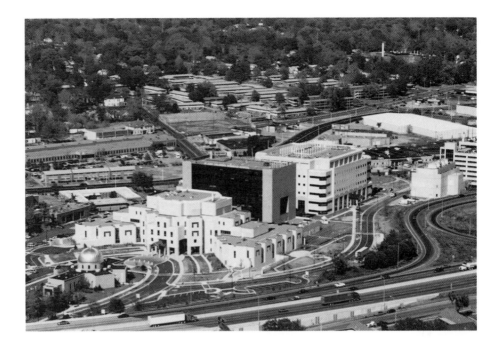

taining space equal to the size of a football field, this high-tech facility has
allowed the hospital to move into new areas of exploring problems encountered
by children with inherited and congenital disorders. These areas include the
department of genetics and hematology/oncology's experimental hematology
and bone marrow transplantation divisions.

In early 1992, construction began on the newest addition to St. Jude's
facilities. Built on the site of the original star-shaped structure, St. Jude's Patient
Care Center was designed to enhance the comfort of patients and families while
further improving standards of care by consolidating patient care services under
one roof. The additional space allowed the hospital to expand certain programs,
such as the bone marrow transplant program, gene therapy and rehabilitation.
Additionally, the new facility contains more space for patients to play, have fun
and try to retain some normalcy in their lives, with three outpatient play rooms,
two inpatient play rooms and a learning center. The 200,000-square-foot facility also features 62 enlarged inpatient rooms, an increase of 14 from the
previous facility, each with a specialized air-filtering system to filter 99.97
percent of all particles in the air.

The basement level of the four-floor terraced facility houses the hospital's primary pharmacy, as well as providing space for behavioral medicine's
division of psychology, the hospital's business offices, public relations, volunteer services, supply processing, delivery and linen services, an employee
fitness center, and medical records storage. An underground parking garage

with space for 50 vehicles helps protect outpatients from extremes of weather.

The ambulatory care unit, with its 33 exam rooms, four consultation rooms, isolation unit and medicine room (where children can watch private television sets as they receive chemotherapy), is housed on the first floor. An expanded outpatient clinic features larger and more comfortable examination, treatment and waiting areas. Also, to ease the unavoidable waiting periods between appointments, families and children have access to libraries, activity rooms and quiet rooms. Pastoral care, a gift shop and a chapel are also on this level.

The second floor holds 40 inpatient rooms, each with an adjoining parent room. The inpatient care floors offer important amenities for patients whose therapy requires longer stays: laundry rooms, private bath facilities for parents, and views overlooking outdoor and lobby areas The third floor houses eight intensive and intermediate care beds and the hospital's first complete surgical suite. A satellite pharmacy on each floor speeds the delivery of medications.

The fourth floor contains a new type of facility for St. Jude. Eight patient rooms and 4,000 square feet of laboratory space comprise the gene therapy unit and bone marrow transplant center. "These labs are specialized labs," says Donna Rill, laboratory supervisor, hematology-oncology. "Just one of the differences is that anyone entering these labs will have to 'gown up' in surgical scrubs and overshoes." The laboratories also meet new Food and Drug Administration guidelines for bone marrow transplantation and gene manipulation.

"What will be done in the gene and cell therapy laboratories will be more in the way of actual, ongoing developmental research where we'll be investigating how best to handle the cells," comments Dr. Nienhuis. "These are not research laboratories in the usual sense — they are clinical application laboratories. They will be used to take what we have learned in the research laboratories about the manipulation of cells or genes, as the case may be, and apply it directly to patient care in an appropriate context."

Development of the cell and gene therapy facility responds to the increasing complexity of bone marrow processing and gene therapy, allowing for new avenues of research that could quickly impact patient care. Because laboratory space is located adjacent to inpatient rooms, materials such as bone marrow cells or peripheral blood cells can be taken from the patients, transported to the lab, manipulated and then returned to the patient, all within the space of a few feet. Dr. Nienhuis says, "The unique advantage we have is that we've been able to design things in the very best way in new space, and design them for children."

More than 1,200 people attended the dedication ceremony of St. Jude Children's Research Hospital's Patient Care Center on October 7, 1994, held during ALSAC's 37th Annual Convention in Memphis. First Lady Hillary Rodham Clinton delivered the keynote address, continuing the tradition of White House participation in St. Jude dedications. Switching from her prepared remarks, she said, "One cannot tour this hospital without being reminded of the unlimited capacity of individual men and women to do things that enhance the human condition. You can feel the sense of hope that permeates this hospital as opposed to other hospitals." Inpatient and ambulatory care patients were moved into the building in the spring of 1995.

Renovation of the 1975 tower completes St. Jude's expansion program. Seventh floor inpatient rooms have been converted to two gene therapy production laboratories and administrative offices. The sixth floor was renovated for occupancy by biostatistics, hematology offices and other offices. The fifth floor is shared by laboratory medicine and pathology. Laboratory medicine also shares space on the fourth floor with infectious diseases. The third floor is occupied by molecular pharmacology.

A large, bright, modern cafeteria at ground level connects the Danny Thomas Research Tower and the 1975 tower. From the start, the hospital cafeteria has been an important meeting place where staff, patients and families intermingle. Since patients, doctors, scientists, staff and volunteers all share the same cafeteria, it's a lively place. Ph.D.s can see the patients they help through their basic research — a very real reminder of what their work is all about.

Through all of the growth and expansion, holding onto the family feeling that initially characterized St. Jude has been a major challenge, as Dr. Mauer said in 1975. Yet despite the increase in staff and personnel, the hospital still retains a personal atmosphere. There is a sense of almost a parent's pride in the progress that has been made, and that has been intentional.

In 1985, Joyce Miller, mother of patient Michelle Miller, described the atmosphere at St. Jude this way: "We've been in lots of hospitals, but St. Jude is completely different. I'm amazed at the way the hospital staff loves and cares for the kids. They care about the parents, too. When it happens to your child, it happens to you. This caring has helped pull us through." Another parent, Ron Galvin, father of neuroblastoma patient Jason, says, "The place just puts its arms around you. There is just a bond between our family and St. Jude Hospital that will always be there." In the words of Dr. Greg McDonald, DDS, whose daughter Kasi died at 2 from neuroblastoma, "St. Jude is a unique place in that the whole staff treats the family as well as the patient."

And the staff has similar feelings about St. Jude. Lisa Walters, a pharmacokinetics research nurse, says, "People ask me how I can work at St. Jude, but I can't think of working anywhere else. The times that sustain me are when the patients smile and hug me. The children are just like Silly Putty, they bounce back. I feel good knowing that maybe I have helped them just a little bit." And there is more to learning than what is found in the laboratory results and clinical studies. "The children and their parents teach us a lot here," says Torrey Sandlund, M.D. "They teach us how to face adversity. They also teach us never to give up. They never give up, so we certainly can't give up in supporting them."

Dr. Raymond K. Mulhern, Ph.D. director of behavioral medicine, says, "Even my best work at St. Jude is humbled by the courage and perseverance of any of our children." And Dr. Andrew Walter, hematologist/oncologist, whose specialty is brain tumors, says, "Personally, it's a privilege to work closely with these families who are going through probably the most terrifying process a parent can go through. I feel privileged that they let me become part of that process, and I try to do what I can to help."

Danny Thomas summed up all of the feeling about St. Jude's effect on

On a cold, windy day, Danny Thomas delivers the keynote speech dedicating the ALSAC-Danny Thomas Pavilion. From left in this Nov. 3, 1982 photo are Ed Barry, Rose Marie Thomas, Bud Rashid, Fred P. Gattas, Sr., Danny, Dr. Mauer and Msgr. Paul Clunan.

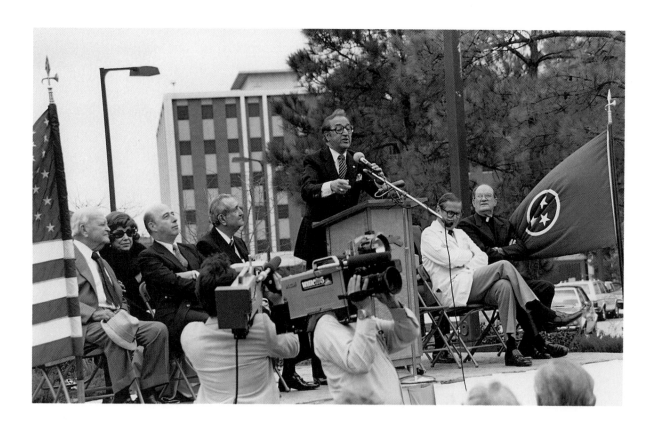

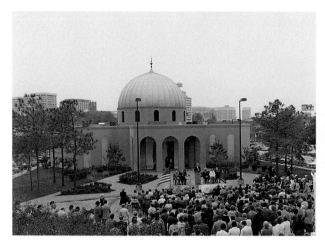

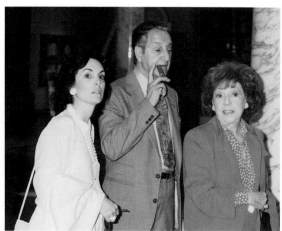

(Left) The ALSAC-Danny Thomas Pavilion was dedicated on Nov. 3, 1982.

(Right) Terre, Danny and Rose Marie Thomas check progress of interior construction at the pavilion during June 1985 visit. The pavilion was built with separate funds given by Arab Americans rather than from hospital donations. It contains the crypt where Danny is now buried.

the people who enter its doors when he said, "The language of love is spoken fluently here at St. Jude."

The smallest major structure on the St. Jude campus is perhaps the most memorable. It is the burial site of the man responsible for creating the hospital that has meant so much to so many. Built from the private donations of ALSAC members, the Danny Thomas/ALSAC Pavilion, like the original hospital, was constructed in the shape of a star, with five alcoves surrounding a rotunda. The star shape symbolizes the far-reaching scope of ALSAC's and St. Jude's work. Designed in the tradition of Middle Eastern architecture, the pavilion's most impressive feature is a gold dome, patterned after the Dome of the Rock in Jerusalem.

Aside from the physical beauty of the building, its most significant aspect is the fact that it was constructed with funds raised exclusively from the board and the Arab-American community and presented to the hospital as their gift. In addition, the Memorial Garden that faces the tomb of Danny Thomas was a gift from the Thomas family and individual board members. While the hospital now has the responsibility of maintaining these facilities, no money donated for St. Jude Children's Research Hospital went into their construction.

Opened in September 1985, the pavilion presents the history of Danny Thomas, St. Jude Children's Research Hospital and ALSAC in a moving display of photographs, audio-visuals and memorabilia. Four of its five alcoves are each devoted to a different aspect of St. Jude's history. One tells the story of ALSAC, its board members and its fund-raising efforts. Danny's career as an entertainer occupies another alcove, complete with the Emmy Awards he received for his role in the *Make Room for Daddy* television show. Another alcove showcases Danny's awards, trophies, honorary degrees, and medals, including the

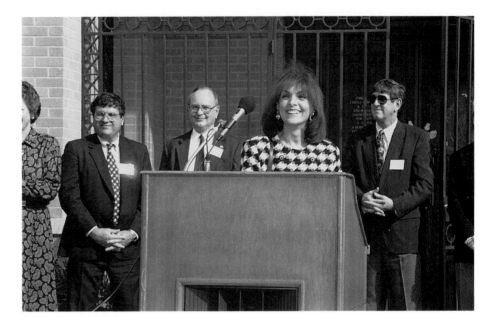

In November 1992, Terre Thomas delivers the dedication address for the Danny Thomas Memorial Garden in front of the crypt where Danny lies. The gardens were a gift of the Danny Thomas family and the Board of Directors.

Congressional Gold Medal of Honor he received for his humanitarian efforts. The patients and the research work conducted at the hospital are the subject of a fourth alcove. A non-denominational chapel and meeting room make up the fifth alcove. A massive mahogany carving of the Last Supper, which Danny commissioned for his home in Beverly Hills, is the focal point of the chapel. This beautiful wood carving hung in Danny's dining room for many years, but he felt it was destined to be in the Pavilion. His wife, Rose Marie, shipped it to Memphis after Danny's death. Thomas is buried in a crypt that backs up to the chapel.

The words of Bishop Daniel Buechlein of the Roman Catholic Diocese of Memphis captured the significance of Danny's interment on the hospital's grounds. "Indeed, his place of rest promises that he will be an immemorial reminder and symbol of the power of prayer of one single person, the power of prayer when all seems hopeless." Danny will be ever-present as the hospital continues to expand to meet the needs of future generations of children.

And expand it will. According to Richard C. Shadyac, ALSAC-St. Jude Board members have already authorized a new long-range planning committee, in conjunction with Dr. Nienhuis and himself, to investigate the possibility that $250 million may be needed for future facilities. "It will happen because we cannot stand still," Shadyac says. "The only way we'll ever do the work of Danny's dream is by growing. And as long as children are dying, we have an obligation."

When faced with the prospect of raising the tremendous amount of money associated with another large expansion, Shadyac is undaunted. "This project belongs to St. Jude," he says, "and he provides."

Inventing A Better Mousetrap

Over the years, ALSAC has become a leader in innovative fund raising. If an idea will help St. Jude and if it's ethical, moral and legal, we'll test it. If it works, we'll run with it.

— **Ruth Ann Skaff, Director of Special Projects**

ALSAC can attribute its thriving growth, in part, to the fact that its staff has not copied fund-raising programs from other national charities. Rather, at each major crossroads in its history, ALSAC has dared to be different. ALSAC has continually explored new and more creative ways of diversifying its fund-raising efforts, and by so doing it has repeatedly exceeded its prior year's performance. This means that, in its relatively short history, ALSAC has been able to surpass the goals it has set for itself. Marie Maddox, mother of St. Jude patient Hollie Maddox, expresses the typical gratitude felt by all St. Jude families when she says, "My daughter has a better cure rate because five years ago someone gave money to help the medicine and the finances and the research at St. Jude."

For many years, ALSAC was dependent on direct mail for most of its funds. ALSAC's direct mail campaigns were initiated in 1958 when Mike Tamer asked his friend Robert J. O'Brian, who had been handling the printing for Tamer's wholesale business, to set up a mailing program for ALSAC's mailing list of members of the Arab-American community. Together the two men, neither of whom had any experience with direct mail, set up a mail program inviting people to become "Founding Fathers" of St. Jude by sending in $1,000 to help equip one of the wings to be built at the hospital. The response to this appeal led Tamer and O'Brian to consider a larger and broader mail appeal. Their first mailing went to 25,000 potential donors in 1960.

In 1961, O'Brian's firm set up a direct mail program for St. Jude and put up $275,000 for the first few years funding. His firm handled virtually the entire operation — copy, art work, printing, mailing, mailing lists, acknowledgments and record-keeping. Within two years, ALSAC had returned the seed

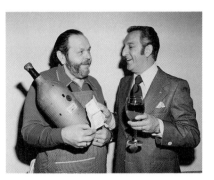
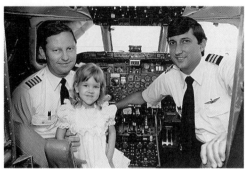

money and a large number of contributions were pouring in.

As reflected in all its fund-raising efforts, ALSAC utilized its direct mail program in diverse and innovative ways. In July 1969, major contributors began receiving updates on the hospital and ALSAC through a newsletter that originated from the direct mail program. Three years later, a sweepstakes program began, with a drawing from a barrel holding 300,000 stubs. When the last drawing was held in 1982, a giant, motor-driven barrel had been built to hold the more than 8,000,000 entries received from each mailing.

In spite of the overt success of the direct mail program, ALSAC's professional staff determined that a direct mail position on the NEO staff would provide more effective mailing strategies and a better cost-per-dollar-raised ratio. In 1981, after a detailed presentation to a special advisory committee of the board by Bud Rashid and members of his staff — Bill Kirwen, Dennis Morlok and Paul Parham — the board approved the transfer of the direct mail program from O'Brian's firm to the new mail appeals department at the National Executive Office. The number of mailings for the previous year had topped 50 million pieces, with receipts in excess of $12 million. More than 2 million active donor names were turned over to the national office. For many years, the direct mail program had been the single largest source of revenue for the hospital. The mail appeals department built on this record. By the end of its first year of operation, even with the director of communications doubling as the interim director of mail appeals, it had decreased expenses by almost half. In the first year under Joe Kachorek, ALSAC's first professional direct mail marketing expert, modern direct mail techniques, elimination of the sweepstakes and reduction of prospect mailing brought in $10.3 million at a cost of only $2.6 million. From 1982 until 1995, the direct mail program grew dramatically.

Mail appeals became ALSAC's first department to top the $30 million mark in total revenue in a single year with a record-breaking $31,003,451 in fiscal year 1994. This represented a 10 percent increase over the previous year and growth of almost 40 percent over the previous five years. The mail appeals department acquired 370,000 new donors in fiscal year 1994, or almost 17 percent more than the previous year, totaling approximately 1.5 million direct mail donors. The average acquisition gift also increased from $15.72 in fiscal year to $17.02 in fiscal year 94.

In June 1995, the direct mail program was combined with the television department to form a new department, the national direct marketing department, under senior vice president Aggie Alexander. Radio acquisition of donors is still separate, but all followup mailing and donor cultivation is now under this new department. In its first year of consolidated operations, the direct mail and the television mail program raised a new record of more than $70 million. Continuing the emphasis on market testing, the National Direct Marketing Department has found that offering direct mail donors an opportunity to use their credit cards works just as well on direct mail appeals as it has for many years with television acquired donors. Concurrently, expenses are being reduced by even greater emphasis on sound business practices, including increasing the vendor base and competitive bidding of all packages.

ALSAC has relied on radio and television for public education since its beginnings, sending out public service announcements as early as 1958. These PSAs provided information about local fund-raising events or about the hospital, but were not in themselves fund-raising appeals. ALSAC began using these media for direct fund-raising efforts only in the late 1960s.

Credit for the first fund-raising radiothon for St. Jude is given to Jacquie Simo for her 1968 Detroit event. Even though St. Paul, Minnesota, and St. Louis, Missouri, radio stations have claims to earlier events, this was the first

(Left) Tony Amores and his father pose for photo used in ALSAC's 1984 Combined Federal Campaign materials. The CFC is conducted by the federal government among civilian and military employees world wide, and is one of the lowest cost fund raising programs ALSAC has.

(Right)Filming at St. Jude always draws spectators. Here a patient gets a close view of monitor during 1987 taping in the original building's waiting room.

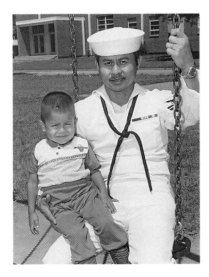

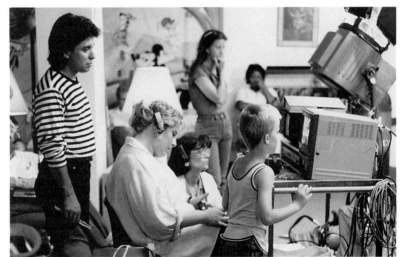

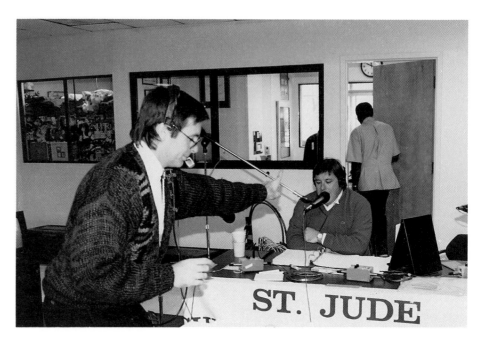

Atlanta's Rhubarb Jones broadcasts live from the lobby of St. Jude during the first Country Cares For St. Jude Kids country music network radiothon in 1989. In 1990, Country Cares went to a mix of local DJ and taped celebrity songs, endorsements and patient stories, becoming one of ALSAC's most successful fund raisers by 1996.

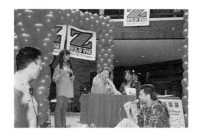

Billy Ray Cyrus dropped in on Z93.9 FM's Country Cares radiothon in Glendale, Calif. Like many of these radiothons, it was a remote broadcast from a shopping mall. All of the radio time and the talent of the local celebrities and the national stars is donated at no cost to St. Jude.

event solely for St. Jude. The daughter of Ethel Bekolay Horste, one of ALSAC's original board members, Simo spent several years developing the materials needed to train volunteers and conduct similar events in other cities. These radiothons were run on a local basis by regional directors and their staffs, or by local chapters and third-party volunteers working for St. Jude. With their inherent need for many volunteers to answer telephones, tabulate pledges, send out acknowledgments, and do all the other physical actions before, during and after the event, radiothons required a large amount of staff time, limiting the number that could be held in a year. In the early years, the regional representatives tried to book radiothons on the largest station in a market, regardless of the station's format. It was soon noticed that country music stations seemed to raise the most money for the hospital. All of this ultimately led to the highly successful national *Country Cares for St. Jude Kids®* program.

Randy Owen of the musical group Alabama was the originator of and is heavily involved in the *Country Cares for St. Jude Kids®* radio campaign, one of ALSAC's fastest-growing fund-raising projects. Alabama had been a donor to St. Jude Children's Research Hospital from the start of its success in the early 1980s. Then when Owen had a chance meeting with Danny Thomas in Nashville, he resolved to do more. He challenged the country music industry to join him, resulting in the Country Cares program.

Begun in 1989, *Country Cares For St. Jude Kids®* is carried by hundreds of radio stations across the country. Stations air one- and two-day radiothons using prerecorded solicitations, endorsements and special music by country music stars. The program has grown from $1.5 million pledged the first year to more than $10.8 million in 1995. Country radio stations in New York, Washington, Tampa, Chicago, Dallas, Los Angeles, Seattle, Nashville and Memphis, among a total of 119 cities.

ALSAC took a far more cautious approach to television due to the cost of establishing a national telethon network. ALSAC's first concentrated entry into telethons came in 1976, when Al Toler implemented a limited test of a format using video-taped entertainment segments from a Norfolk, Virginia, local telethon produced by the Norfolk chapter and Jess Duboy, a television advertising personality. This telethon's amateur entertainment acts were taped and then sent to other areas in ALSAC's Southern Region where they were integrated into live, local productions.

The test showed potential, and Danny Thomas reluctantly entered the telethon arena a year later, when he hosted his first live, local telethon with Kate Jackson as co-host. The five hour Los Angeles telecast in 1977 raised $338,664. When the results were in, Danny said, "I can't remember why I never wanted to do this." Results were even better when ALSAC's director of communications edited the show's tapes to two-and-a-half hours of entertainment that was then used for more than 20 local telethons across the country. These local telethons were put on by ALSAC's regional directors in communities where they found a television station willing to sell them time, enough local entertainers to go on air, and volunteers to answer telephones and handle all of the myriad details that go into putting on a successful live show.

Although the results were impressive, this system was labor-intensive and precarious, relying as it did on shipping tapes from one region to another. The potential for disaster was always there, and it almost happened. In 1979 Dave Long, the New England Region director, called Memphis frantically on a Saturday morning to report that a janitor at the station that was going to air his telethon on Sunday had inadvertently erased all the tapes. Only the rapid response of ALSAC's director of development Bill Kirwen and director of communications Paul Parham, and the generosity of a Delta Airlines pilot flying to Boston who put the five large cans of tape beside his seat got a duplicate set of tapes to Long in time for his broadcast.

By 1980, the success of the local telethons had overtaxed the regional offices' ability to organize and service them. Again ALSAC's innovative thinking was called on to open a new avenue for solicitations. Live local segments and pure entertainment segments were discarded in favor of a fully scripted, video-taped special, produced by the Russ Reid Company of Pasadena, California.

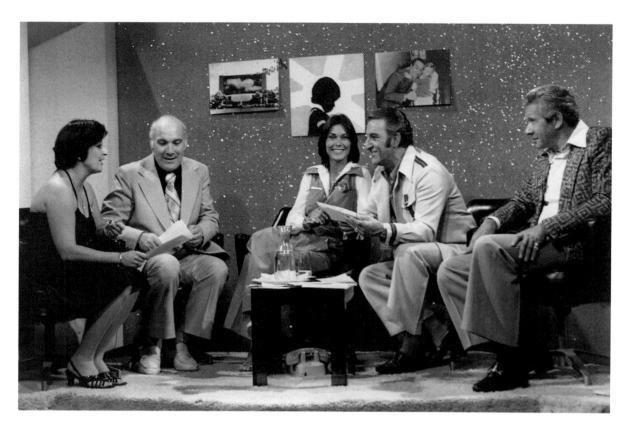

Danny and Kate Jackson co-hosted the first Los Angeles telethon in 1979. ALSAC took a very cautious approach to television because of the huge expenses associated with a live, national hook up. For a short time, the entertainment segments from this live telethon, then one in New York in 1980, and finally one in Las Vegas in 1981 were extracted and used as inserts in live telethons held in a small number of local markets at later times. In 1982, ALSAC began its current system of completely taping a special and then airing it in many markets all over America throughout the year.

This special featured the hospital staff, patients and selected entertainers. In October 1981 the test of this new concept in television fund raising for St. Jude began when *Let the Children Live*, with Michael Landon and Dianna Canova as co-hosts, aired in seven test markets, beginning with Spokane, Washington. The show actually was three hours long, but the first two hours were repeated as hours four and five to make it a five-hour show .

Viewers responded compassionately to the up-close and personal look at the people of St. Jude, calling their pledges in to a professional national telephone answering service. The show began airing in markets all over America in December, and by June 30, 1982, it had been shown in more than 85 markets, more than quadrupling the number of showings and at far less staff time than in the past. In addition to generating funds, this special provided a much wider audience with information on the life-saving work of doctors and scientists at St. Jude and the experiences of patients and their parents.

The tremendous increase in its broadcast fund-raising programs led to the creation of a department of broadcasting in 1981 to handle both radio and television. Since radiothons remained primarily a regional tool, supervision of radio was soon returned to the associate director of development who supervised the regional offices. Since the adoption of a taped format, five-hour, three-hour, one-hour and half-hour versions of programs with Danny and Marlo Thomas as host and hostess have been tested and aired. The results showed the one-hour television special was the most effective. In 1991, 60-second and 120-second commercials were launched, allowing the hospital to penetrate the large cable networks. From 1988 to 1994, the television marketing department, successor to the broadcasting department, went from raising $12 million a year to nearly $30 million. And with experience, most of the functions originally handled by an outside agency such as media buying and placement, operation of the donor base and supervision of the mail follow-up program, were taken over by the television department. Now 60 to 70 percent of St. Jude placements are in prime time.

A Gift of Love, co-hosted by Marlo Thomas and actor John Goodman, went on the air in 1992 and continues to be effective after 48 months, longer than any other show about the hospital's life-saving work. *Race Against Time*, a one-hour docudrama also featuring Marlo Thomas and John Goodman as hosts, began airing in the spring of 1994. *For Our Children,* featuring footage from previous shows with updated patient stories, went on the air in 1995. Plans call for a new one-hour television special every two to three years, with new commercials each year.

With Danny Thomas' strong business and personal ties to Hollywood, celebrity events were a natural fund-raising theme from the beginning. After the success of two shows held in Memphis in 1955 and 1957, a series of Shower of Star shows were staged there during the 1960s and into the 1970s. Wayne Newton, Tennessee Ernie Ford, Sammy Davis Jr, Paul Anka and Frank Sinatra were among the many stars who appeared on these shows. Top names in show business loved and respected Danny and responded personally to his dream.

The shows initiated a tradition of galas and theme parties at several chapters with each creating their own signature events. The Inspiration Ball was just such an event, founded by the city director of the Greater Detroit Chapter of ALSAC, Ethel Bekolay Horste, a member of the original ALSAC Board of Directors, in honor of her daughter Jacquie, who herself had successfully fought illness. In Miami, the Miracle Ball, first held in 1961, was founded by Anthony and Genevieve Abraham. Tom Abraham continues his parents event.

In 1979, Rose Marie Thomas produced the most successful fund-raising dinner ALSAC had ever had to that time, raising $426,000. Almost 1,500 people contributed a minimum of $125 each to attend the event, with Phyllis McGuire and oil magnate Mike Davis contributing $100,000. It was McGuire's third such donation, and the pharmacology division of St. Jude is dedicated to her generosity.

The following year, Rose Marie's gala, billed as "Sinatra Sings: A Night in Italy," gathered 2,000 admirers of Frank Sinatra at the Century Plaza Hotel in Beverly Hills to celebrate Frank and Barbara Sinatra's fourth wedding anniversary. A million dollars was raised that night for St. Jude. George Burns, Marcia and Neil Diamond, Bob and Dolores Hope, Lucille Ball, Carol Burnett, Jack Lemmon, Liza Minelli, Jan Murray, Joey Bishop, Steve Lawrence and Eydie Gorme, James W. Near and R. David Thomas of Wendy's International Inc. are just a few of the many celebrity benefactors attending this event over the years.

In March 1996, Rose Marie and co-chairs Marlo, Terre and Tony Thomas produced the 16th annual Rose Marie Thomas Gala Dinner featuring an evening with singer Tony Bennett and Roseanne at the Beverly Hilton Hotel. With the largest single gift ever made to this event — a $1 million pledge from movie mogul David Geffen — a total of $2.1 million was raised for the hospital, the most successful single event in ALSAC history. And surprisingly, although the St. Jude Foundation of California has technically been listed as the sponsor, it has been Rose Marie, Janet Roth and a small group of friends volunteering their help who have actually made this dinner the most impressive charity event on the Los Angeles social calendar.

Other significant dinners include the Marguerite Piazza Annual Gala, an event sponsored in Memphis by the former Metropolitan opera star, and the Miracle Rock concerts produced by Tom Abraham in Miami since 1989, featuring such performers as Buddy Guy, Whitney Houston, Neil Diamond, Kenny G., Tina Turner and Bette Midler. In 1996, John Lattanzio, partner in Wall Street's Steinhardt Partners, and Elizabeth Larson, managing director of Soros Fund Management, were honored with the Michael F. Tamer Award, ALSAC's highest commendation. They led a blue chip committee of Wall Street

(Left) Danny Thomas and Dr. Joseph V. Simone get their instructions during taping of the 1987 St. Jude television special. This shot on the hospital's 7th floor inpatient area was typical of the unusual use some parts of the hospital got during these filming sessions.

(Right) Marguerite Piazza performs at her Marguerite Piazza Gala for St. Jude, one of several annual formal benefits held each year.

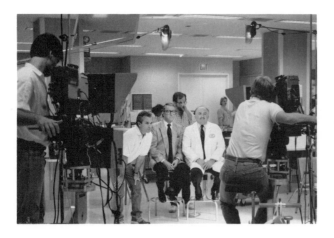

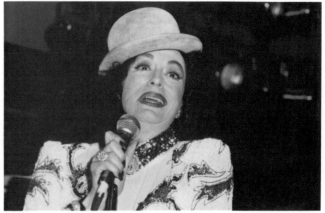

financiers in raising $3.6 million with a series of dinners in New York City over a five-year period. Their campaign established 24 new research laboratories in the Danny Thomas Research Tower.

ALSAC's most remarkable innovation in the field of fundraising, however, may be the establishment and operation of its own unique telemarketing program. Bill Kirwen's Community Development Program of 1977 cited earlier has now evolved into the telemarketing arm of ALSAC. In addition to focusing on schools and small communities, the ALSAC approach is unusual in that its telephone power is not used for direct appeals for money but rather to recruit event chairmen. Following the initial test in two regions, telemarketing sections were established in each regional office. After phenomenal growth, operations were consolidated into two large telephone centers, one in Memphis and the other in New Albany, Indiana, near Louisville. ALSAC calls them its Volunteer Service Centers (VSC I and VSC II). Under the guidance of the telemarketing support department at the National Executive Office, the VSCs administer telemarketing programs that cover the entire country.

ALSAC's telemarketing events start with Volunteer Service Center staff calls to recruit volunteer event chair people. These volunteers then run telemarketing fund-raising events for St. Jude such as bike-a-thons, Math-A-Thons® , Saddle-Up for St. Jude, and Trivia Challenges, using materials and guidelines supplied by the National Executive Office. Following the event, the donations are sent to Memphis for accounting. After verification, T-shirts and other incentives earned by the event participants are shipped to the chairman for distribution. While there is no direct face-to-face interaction between ALSAC staff and the volunteers, a series of regular telephone calls helps create a personal bond between the volunteer, the hospital and the ALSAC staff.

According to Marilyn Elledge, director of VSC I in Memphis, she and Ron Casabella, director of VSC II, recruit more than 25,000 volunteer chairmen each year by telephone, using only 120 seasonal staff members to do the calling. On average, each event raises $1,000.

Print and video materials produced by ALSAC's communications department have helped ALSAC meet and surpass its fund-raising goals over the years. ALSAC provides each coordinator recruited to conduct a telemarketing event with all of the materials — coordinator guides, sponsor forms, posters, video tapes, etc. — needed from start to finish. Functioning like an in-house advertising and public relations agency, the communications department writes, designs and oversees production of these materials, ensuring that they are on hand each year when the campaign starts. In addition, national public service announcements for radio, TV and magazines; public education films; the quarterly ALSAC News newspaper; quarterly Partners In Hope tabloid, brochures; pamphlets; and the combined annual report of the hospital and ALSAC are all produced and distributed by this department, which has been a consistent winner of national, regional and local advertising and public relations awards for its materials created in support of ALSAC's fund-raising efforts. The titles of the 15-minute informational films produced through the years capture the essence of St. Jude's mission: *Half Sung Songs* (1975), *A Child of Us All* (1978), *A Family Album* (1983), *That They Shall Live* (1987), and *Children of the Dream* (1991).

Danny Thomas thoughts at the end of *Half Sung Songs*, pinpoint the reasons behind the continuing efforts to tell St. Jude's message to all who will listen:

> There are still children whose "song is half sung . . . unfurnished rooms . . . poems begun that end too soon." Each time I visit our haven of mercy in Memphis, Tennessee, I am told of brighter tomorrows for the children of this world, a tomorrow whose bounds are limitless. Perhaps among them is one who will conquer the universe,. . . or find a way to calm another's fears. Perhaps among these precious children is the one who would find a cure for the suffering of them all.

More impressive than the sheer numbers of volunteers are the individuals themselves. Many volunteers, most of whom have never visited St. Jude, go "above and beyond" in raising money for the hospital. These outstanding volunteers commonly cite persistence, hard work and the generous spirit of their communities as key ingredients that make their own particular fund-raiser shine. Math-A-Thon®, one of the most successful community-based fund-raising programs, is now held in more than 10,000 schools across the country. It was created by Fran Madrid and first tried in her Mid-Atlantic Region in 1978. Children in kindergarten through ninth grade who want to participate in the program are provided with special Funbooks filled with math problems appropriate to the child's grade level. The children solicit pledges for donations from family, friends and neighbors based on the number of math problems they complete. In 1993, almost 400,000 students were a part of Math-A-Thon, bringing in more than $12 million in pledges.

To Marie Walton of Hamilton, Ohio, a teacher and mother, the appeal of a St. Jude Math-A-Thon was obvious. "I love kids and want to work with

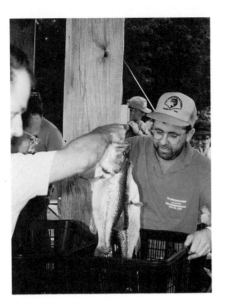 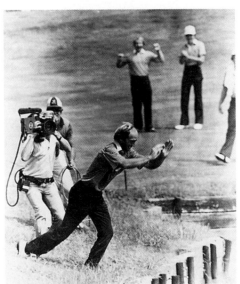

(Left) The St. Jude Bass Classic in Mississippi is one of several fishing tournaments held for the hospital. Here one team's catch is weighed in May 1992.

(Right) PGA pro Jerry Pate takes a jump in the lake on the 18th hole after winning the 1981 Danny Thomas Memphis Classic, now called the FedEx St. Jude Classic.

kids. These things go with being a teacher. They also go with being a mother," she explains.

Marie first received information on a St. Jude Math-A-Thon in the mail at a time when her school district's math scores were not as high as its reading scores. A Math-A-Thon seemed to offer a double benefit: "I felt like this was a worthy cause and I wanted to do something that would focus on math."

Marie was able to raise an astounding $44,000 over the course of two Math-A-Thons at Hopewell Elementary School. "After the first year, I was shocked by how much money I raised," Marie laughs. "I got the teachers pumped and they helped me get the students pumped up." Information Marie received about St. Jude patients helped motivate her to organize the Math-A-Thons. "I would read these things about these children and I would get tears in my eyes."

She says she encountered no resistance in the community to raising money for a charity not considered "local." "St. Jude, the way I see it, is for children in every community. If someone here has a need, they can go there. They accept anybody from any community," Marie explains.

Floridian Kathy Ayers runs the Twin Pines Stable outside Orlando. She has organized three Saddle-Up Trail Rides for St. Jude since 1992. Hers is one of the largest trail rides, and her work begins the year before the event, soliciting donations of food, prizes and raffle items from area merchants. "I try to get anything and everything donated," Kathy says.

Approximately 100 to 150 horse riders participate in her 10-mile trail ride each year. The rides cross land belonging to several property owners around Orlando, from all of whom Kathy must secure permission to use before the ride, not always and easy task. "Trail bosses," experienced riders Kathy knows, mark the trail the day before the Saddle-Up and lead groups of riders on the trail. Extra side events and the pledges of the riders have helped raise nearly $21,000 for St. Jude over the course of Kathy's three Saddle-Ups.

This is especially remarkable in light of the fact that not only has Kathy never been to St. Jude, she also doesn't know anyone who has. She was recruited over the telephone by Volunteer Service Center staffers. Kathy is motivated to organize the Saddle-Ups because, "It's for the children. It's for a good cause. All the work and effort is well worth it when you see these children [on videos and in print materials provided by the hospital]."

Many of the Saddle-Up participants are retirees who travel around the country going on trail rides. They begin collecting sponsors for the following year's ride as soon as the current year's ride is over. "They'll be somewhere and say, 'Hey, in April I'm going to be in Indiana in a trail ride for St. Jude. Do you want to sponsor me?' " Chris Thomas of Martinsville, Indiana, explains. As a nurse, animal lover and owner of Springcliffe Farm, Chris says the attitude of the kids at St. Jude and the hospital's fiscal responsibility are what keep her interested. "Every dollar we can give the children that will help make them more comfortable or have a day that is pain free, they're appreciative of. It's a good feeling."

ALSAC's fund-raising efforts follow potential donors from the "cradle to the grave." With programs aimed at toddlers, senior citizens and every age in between, ALSAC's broad range of activities cover every aspect of society. Furthermore the VSCs have targeted a diverse array of local organizations

(Left) Coors Brewing Company employees give all patients a Halloween pumpkin in 1994. Coors sponsors the St. Jude Halloween promotion.

(Right) Patients are often asked to model the incentive prizes for posters used to promote ALSAC telemarketing events. Here long term survivors Ann Brinkmann and Brian Doyle show off the 1995 prizes for Saddle Up horse back riding events.

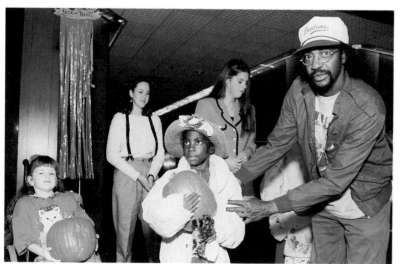

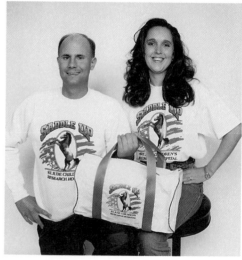

throughout the country as venues for innovative and creative fund-raising programs to increase public awareness, foster community support and raise needed funds.

All ALSAC's telemarketing fund-raising programs depend on both volunteers and the behind-the-scenes support staff of the ALSAC National Executive Office. People like ALSAC's Production Center employees are key factors in ensuring ALSAC's success.

The Production Center is ALSAC's distribution hub, receiving, storing and shipping all the campaign materials associated with the telelemarketing programs. Using the latest technology, such as bar coding of outgoing parcels, the center's eight-employee staff assembles and ships all the materials needed to run the telemarketing events. This includes program kit materials such as sponsor forms, sign-up sheets, money-return envelopes and sample T-shirts; incentives, such as T-shirts and tote bags; and awards, including calculators, VCRs and TVs. In 1995 the center handled approximately 120,000 shipments, an increase of almost 500 percent from the its shipment numbers in the early 1980s. According to former Production Center manager Larry Medler, even as recently as 1992, "if we could get out 350 orders a day, that was a full day's work, and that was doing good. Now [1996] we can run 1,200 with no problem."

The Production Center is the last link in the telemarketing chain, and comes into play after the Volunteer Service Centers have completed their recruitment and an event, such as a Math-A-Thon, has been scheduled. "We are sending out the actual kit," says Medler. "We are sending it to volunteers, so if we send them the wrong material, there's a possibility that that chairman will resign. I would say it's very vital to the operation. Once we put our hands on it and fill that T-shirt order or fill that kit order and it goes out the door, the accuracy has to be up as high as it can be."

Most of the participants in ALSAC's telemarketing events are young people and students. Young people have long been a target for ALSAC's fund-raising efforts, starting with the Teen Age Marches of the 1960s. It seems only right that through the years those most easily able to identify with St. Jude's patients have come through with the funds to give these patients another chance. Overall, an estimated 800,000 to 1,000,000 people actively participate in the telemarketing program events conducted for St. Jude Children's Research Hospital each year. For fiscal year 1996, these events raised more than $26 million, a remarkable total in every regard for programs that start with a telephone call.

Runs for St. Jude are also popular. In 1981, Sigma Nu fraternity brothers jogged non-stop the 300 miles from Hattiesburg, Mississippi, to St. Jude, raising $6,000. Volunteers from the St. Jude Affiliate in Peoria, Illinois, run from Memphis to Peoria every summer, raising pledges for the Peoria telethon produced by longtime board member and Peoria Mayor Jim Maloof. In August 1995, runners garnered $326,000 in pledges, giving the event a 14-year total of almost $2 million. And 1996 saw the 19th annual Oak Hall Run for St. Jude in Memphis. The 3-mile run/jog/walk event included more than 3,200 runners, garnering $80,000 for St. Jude. Since the event first began in 1978, it has raised more than $1.5 million for the children of St. Jude and earned race director and founder Bill Levy and his helpers the title of ALSAC's Volunteer Group of the Year for 1994.

Sports have long played a strong role in fundraising for the hospital, with campaigns centered around tennis, football and, most notably, golf. Since 1960, when a check for $600 was delivered from the Memphis professional golf tournament, then named the Memphis Open, St. Jude Children's Research Hospital and golf in Memphis have been closely connected. Renamed the Danny Thomas Memphis Classic and then the Federal Express St. Jude Classic, this Professional Golf Association tournament, sponsored and produced by a separate non-profit organization of Memphis golf lovers, attracts names from both the professional and amateur world of golf. Such notable amateurs as former President Gerald Ford — who hit a hole in one at the tournament the year he left the White House and gave the ball to the hospital to be auctioned — Michael Jordan, Bob Hope and Phil Donahue, as well as professionals including Lee Trevino, have all teed off for St. Jude. As the beneficiary of the FedEx St. Jude Classic, St. Jude received a gift of $755,108 in 1993 from the tournament, players contributions and the PGA Tour Partners Program and Team Charity competition. Since the tournament first chose the hospital as its sole beneficiary in 1970, the hospital has realized more than $5.5 million. More than 1,400 volunteers serve throughout the week of the annual event.

ALSAC itself sponsors amateur golf events with the assistance of its own volunteers. The 4th Annual Roy Clark Celebrity Gala raised $1.1 million in 1995. This event, under chairman Ray Imperial, consists of two celebrity golf tournaments and a celebrity dinner in West Palm Beach, Florida. ALSAC board members Lance Lucibello and Dr. Bob Breit chaired the 6th Annual St. Jude Hospital Celebrity Golf Classic in Medinah, Illinois, in 1995, raising $140,000. Board member V. Reo Campion founded and has produced the Danny Thomas St. Jude Golf Classic at Indian Wood Country Club north of Detroit, raising more than $70,000 in 1995 for a total of $1.7 million in 23 years.

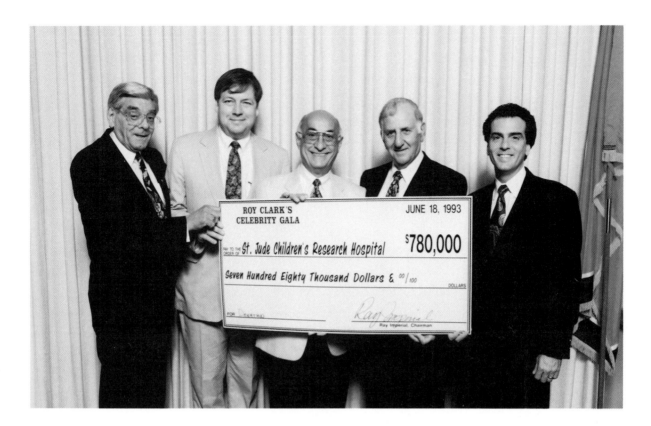

Many local groups hold golf tournaments for St. Jude. One of the largest is the Roy Clark Celebrity Gala in West Palm Beach, Fla. In this 1993 photo, event chairman Ray Imperial in the center presents tournament proceeds to, from left, ALSAC national executive director Dick Shadyac, St. Jude Hospital director Dr. Art Nienhuis, chairman of the St. Jude board Ed Eissey and chairman of the ALSAC board Paul Simon.

With golf classics for amateurs held all over the U.S. featuring thousands of players, spectators and volunteers hitting the courses for St. Jude, the potential of these local tournaments has led to the addition of a new position, director of golf, to ALSAC's field operations department, with Tom Lenz, an experienced golfer and fund-raiser, working to set up new tournaments wherever possible.

Grass-roots fund raising for St. Jude takes all forms, from haunted houses and dinner dances in small towns in Georgia and Massachusetts to such national efforts as the Cool Ghoul-Halloween program, created for retail food establishments across the country in 1993. Refined and renamed the Coors Halloween Promotion in recognition of sponsorship by Coors Brewing Company, the program is aimed at adults. Dave McKee, senior vice president for field operations, sees this program's future lying in the chain marketing accounts where commercial distributors do the whole event and St. Jude gets the net, thereby once again keeping ALSAC's professional staff and fund-raising costs at a minimum.

McKee points out increasing cooperation between the region offices and the Volunteer Service Centers (VSCs) on grass-root events."With the VSC's doing 'pre-calls' [asking for renewals in advance of the event] for Country Cares for the regions, we have had a 10 percent repledge rate." He also cites new region-VSC joint ventures such as *Capture for St. Jude Kids*, a program where the VSC calls into a town and recruits a celebrity jailbird for the event while the region takes care of the event details such as getting a location for the jail, doing the publicity and setting up the collections point for the bail pledges to St. Jude. This example of the type of creative thinking going into grass-roots fund raising pays off. Four tests have averaged $10,000 in 1995, he says. In addition, McKee, who is responsible for all field activities, including the VSCs and the regions, says that the VSCs will test trying to get *Capture for St. Jude Kids* to be a stand-alone project like the bike rides, with a chairman in a small town doing the entire event.

Along with its attention to community fund-rasing drives and individual chapter events, ALSAC also seeks gifts of corporate and foundation dollars, planned giving and large individual bequests, primarily for ALSAC's endowment program. In recent years, these functions have been centralized and now are the responsibility of Richard C. Hackett, senior vice president for endowment and major gifts. Getting to this current structure and policy is a relatively recent development in ALSAC history.

A planned giving department was added in 1978, with Judy Simpson as the first director. Planned giving includes bequests by will, gift annuities,

Another form of support that became popular in the 1980s are runs and walks of various lengths and categories. This is the start of the 1985 Oak Hall Run in Memphis, now one of the largest charity runs in America.

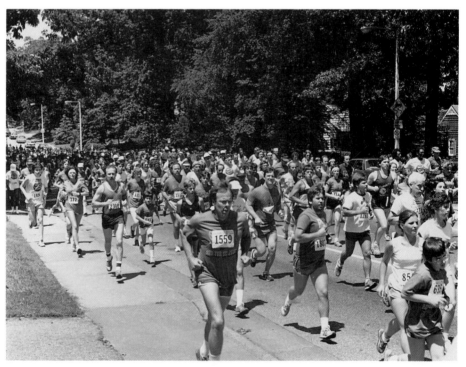

trusts and property donations. Until then, ALSAC had done little to seek income from deferred giving. Gifts from estates came without an active program and brought comparatively little revenue to the hospital. With Simpson and then in 1979 her assistant, Leslie Mason Bailey, the planned giving department started on a course of steady growth, adding new programs through the years. Programs such as estate planning seminars provide a personal service to potential donors while also encouraging them to remember the hospital in their plans. Donor recognition programs such as the Danny Thomas-St. Jude Society, started in 1993 to recognize contributors who have included the hospital in their estate planning, help maintain donor interest.

By 1986, planned giving revenue was $5 million. That grew to more than $20 million in 1995, a growth of more than 300 percent. In 1994, Leslie Mason Bailey returned from other employment to become ALSAC's planned giving director. Her department now has three regional planned giving directors and one associate director, with plans to add offices in Dallas, Chicago and one to cover the East Coast of Florida. Bailey says her main change is a shift of marketing focus since 1993 by re-targeting the potential donor population and preparing materials for them based on their age rather than concentrating on the wealth demographic.

Along with the restructured planned giving program, the major gifts division is concentrating on expanding opportunities in the corporate and foundation arenas, targeting the small business community as well as large corporations and foundations. Hackett sees the biggest trend in his area as the emphasis on corporate fund raising, "going after outright gifts and cause-related marketing programs."

"We show them the consumer would rather do business with a corporation with a conscience," he says. "We treat the corporation as an individual, appealing to their compassion and at the same time to their sense of business." Hackett says the ALSAC approach is to recognize that corporations and the people that comprise them are all different and to treat each corporation differently.

Early on, Danny Thomas had a vision of funding St. Jude Children's Research Hospital in perpetuity through the establishment of an endowment fund. He believed that the hospital should be freed from any uncertainty regarding its financial future, and in 1981, the first endowment campaign was planned. This ultimately led to the establishment of the St. Jude 21st Century Fund, officially launched on June 13, 1991. Based on early planning in the 1980s, today's endowment goals are to raise $250 million by the year 2000.

Dick Shadyac projects earlier success. "We are already beyond our expectations," he says, "and we will attain by the year 2000, probably before, the $250 million figure." After that, he predicts that the board will set another goal of $500 million. To meet these goals, all monies raised from telemarketing events have been earmarked for the endowment fund, and are designated as such in the materials produced for those events.

As Bud Rashid stated during his long tenure as ALSAC's executive director, "The more successful we are, the larger the burden becomes. The more children who survive, the more costly it is going to be for us to keep the institution going because each patient is a patient for life."

Although responsibility for the hospital's continued well-being rests firmly with ALSAC, it is ultimately the American public who has determined the future of St. Jude. The generous donations of time, energy and money from millions of American citizens have fueled ALSAC's every program. Whether received as a $10 individual contribution or a million dollar bequest, the contributions of ALSAC's supporters have made St. Jude's patient care and research advances possible.

Raising the money required for St. Jude's research and patient care is not an easy task, but each year ALSAC continues to generate more funds from the public than ever before to meet the hospital's costs. Approximately 6 million people contribute an average $18 to ALSAC and St. Jude each year. An estimated 1 million volunteers from all parts of America take part in the thousands of bike rides, Math-A-Thons, and other telemarketing fund-raising events; put on dinners, golf tournaments and other chapter activities; and respond to the call for support.

Danny Thomas knew the importance of far-reaching appeal. "I'd rather have a million people give me a dollar than one give me a million," he once said. "That way you've got a million people involved."

Among the early fund-raisers for St. Jude were people who suffered from serious illness. Such a person was Ann Hill of Ashland, Mississippi. Although Ann suffered from a rare disease and was never able to walk, she sold lemonade for St. Jude, raising $1,108 when she was 11 years old to give to Danny when the hospital opened. For her dedication through the years, Ann was named volunteer chairman for the state of Mississippi. She continued to work with Teen Marches and other events, and at her death in 1970 at the age of 25, ALSAC announced that she had help raise almost $150,000 for the hospital.

The Jerry Nicholson Award, the highest tribute that ALSAC pays to a young volunteer, is given annually in honor of a St. Jude patient from Riverside, California, who not only battled leukemia in the early years of St. Jude, but also organized and led fund-raising activities for the hospital. As Danny Thomas wrote in his letters to the award's recipients, "Even in his last months when he knew he wasn't going to make it, Jerry led a 'pints for half-pints' blood donor campaign for St. Jude in Riverside, calling from Memphis to make sure it was going well, even as his own life ebbed away. He was an inspiration to all who knew him."

Individual contributions have come in numbers great and small. Sam Cooper, a Memphian and former president of Humko Products, headed fund-raising drives in Memphis in both 1974 and 1986. The 1974 Mission for Memphis raised a total of $4,200,000 for cancer research at St. Jude and the University of Tennessee Memphis Center for Health Sciences, with Cooper contributing $50,000 to the campaign. Cooper had already committed himself to a $2 million drive for University of Tennessee Memphis cancer research when Danny Thomas asked him to head up a drive to raise $2 million to pay off the costs of St. Jude's new addition. Instead of saying no, Cooper combined the drives, raising the funds in just three-and-a-half months. Cooper had lost a daughter to cancer himself. "One of four families in this country is touched by cancer. If you are not you ought to get down on your knees every night and thank the man upstairs for being so blessed. If you have gone through this ordeal, you have to be as dedicated as you can to prevent someone else from suffering as you did." In 1986, he, along with board members Jack Belz and Fred Smith, headed up the second Mission for Memphis campaign to raise the funds Memphis business had promised if the board would stay in Memphis (as mentioned earlier). In addition to heading these two major capital gift campaigns, Cooper has given years of service to the FedEx St. Jude Golf Classic, the Marguerite Piazza Gala and other Memphis events for St. Jude.

Another Memphian, noted restaurateur John Grisanti, made history in 1979 at an auction of rare old wines when he bid the highest price ever paid for a single bottle of wine. He returned to Memphis and uncorked the bottle at a wine tasting party to benefit the hospital. A gourmet dinner and a sip of wine at $1,400 per person brought $45,000 to St. Jude. In 1980, he broke his previous record by paying $31,000 for a 158-year-old bottle of Chateau Lafite. Nine Memphis businessmen and Grisanti each contributed $3,000 to purchase the wine at auction. Two hundred people paid $200 each to attend a wine-tasting gala, where lots were drawn for the privilege of sipping the rare wine. The hospital received $53,000 from the event.

Entertainers by the hundreds have supported Danny Thomas and St. Jude. As a special bonus to the staff and patients, these celebrities also come to

visit the hospital. Hollywood legend Frank Sinatra, in particular, is one individual who has proven his support for St. Jude throughout the years. The sixth
floor of the hospital's seven-story tower is dedicated to him for his many benefits in St. Jude's name. The seventh floor is dedicated to Ray Kroc of McDonald's
Restaurants, who donated a million dollars of stock to the hospital and whose
restaurant crews dedicated many hours to helping out with telethons and
special fund-raising projects.

Third-party organizations have also long been an important part of
ALSAC's ability to raise the funds needed to support St. Jude, in some cases
years before the hospital was built. Among the earliest was the N. G. Beram
Veterans Association of Boston, which under its commander, Emile Hajar,
formed ALSAC's first chartered chapter. Danny Thomas' acceptance of the Hotel
Employee and Restaurant Employees Union contribution of $250,000 in 1960
began a long history of union support. By 1996, H.E.R.E. had given more than
$2.3 million to St. Jude, and some locals of other unions, like the Fire Fighters
Association Local 1784 in Memphis, have assessed themselves for a monthly
contribution to the hospital from each member. Over the years, the Jaycees,
Fraternal Order of the Eagles, the Ladies Auxiliary of the American Legion,
VFW Auxiliary, VFW, Alpha Delta Kappa, National Beta Club, North American
Benefit Association and numerous other groups have volunteered their support.
Tau Kappa Epsilon Fraternity, Arthur Murray International, the national Catholic
Youth Organization Federation, along with countless other groups and organi-
zations have contributed at their national, regional or local level to the hospital.

All third-party groups are important to the hospital, but the women of
Epsilon Sigma Alpha International, a national service sorority for women from
all walks of life, deserve special recognition as St. Jude's largest single third-
party supporter in terms of dollars raised for the hospital. In 1969, ESA board
member Judy Lester met Danny Thomas and began working to bring ESA and
St. Jude together. Through her efforts Danny was invited to become an honorary sister in ESA. Simultaneously, Jim Maloof, a member of the St. Jude Board
since 1958, was working with ESA's Illinois chapters to involve ESA with St.
Jude. Through their joint efforts St. Jude and ESA formed a partnership for the
children of the world. Judy Lester then conceived the idea for "ESA's Million
Dollar Bike Ride" supporting St. Jude, which coupled a national event with
local rides sponsored by each ESA chapter in 1971. Two years later, when Lester
was elected ESA international president, St. Jude became the first international
project for ESA. ESA has now raised more than $25 million, and the fourth
floor of the ALSAC Tower at the hospital is named in honor of the women of

ESA. In 1996, its 24th year of helping the hospital, ESA raised $2.2 million for St. Jude and in addition pledged to raise $5 million to endow the fourth floor of the Patient Care Center.

Whether through car washes, can recycling, toy drives, auctions, dinners or numerous other events, or through a steady monthly contribution solicited through its mail appeals, St. Jude and ALSAC owe their success to the people who care. As chairman of the ALSAC Board of Directors, Paul Simon addressed these people in the 1993 ALSAC annual report, writing, "As a result of your commitment to helping children overcome catastrophic diseases, a family faced with a child's devastating illness need not be overcome by despair. Instead, thanks to the generosity of people like you, that family can receive a message of hope from the staff of St. Jude Children's Research Hospital."

In the words of Danny Thomas, "Those who have shared my dream of St. Jude Children's Research Hospital owe a special debt to our fellow citizens, for without them this hospital would not exist, and mankind would be the worse for that."

CONQUERING CATASTROPHIC CHILDHOOD DISEASE

When people complain about little everyday problems, I tell them to go to St. Jude to see the little children there.

Linda Wilson, a member of the first group of patients
St. Jude Hospital considered cured, telling her story in 1989 at age 27

Lindsay and Lauren Conner entered the world six weeks before they were due. A year later, in August 1992, their parents, Stan and Susan Conner, were grappling with the fear that they might lose one of the beautiful twins. Lindsay, normally a bright, happy 1-year-old, had lost her appetite and become lethargic. When a visit to her doctor revealed that both her ears were infected, she was sent home with an antibiotic. A few days later, a lump appeared above her left ear; then, a week later, another the size of a golf ball appeared on her cheek. When Lindsay's doctor heard about the appearance of the second lump, he decided to run some tests.

The results revealed acute myeloid leukemia (AML), a stubborn, partic- ularly difficult cancer to heal. Lindsay's grandfather had died from AML earlier that year, after only three weeks of chemotherapy. Having experienced the effects of the disease so recently, Lindsay's parents were terrified for their little girl.

Leukemia is the most common form of cancer in children. The two most common forms of childhood leukemias are acute lymphocytic leukemia (also called acute lymphoblastic leukemia), commonly known as ALL, and acute myelocytic leukemia (also called acute myelogenous leukemia), com- monly known as AML. ALL accounts for 80 percent of the estimated 2,500 new cases of childhood leukemia diagnosed each year in the United States. AML occurs in approximately 18 percent of childhood leukemia cases, with about 500 new pediatric diagnoses annually.

In a child with leukemia, white blood cells in the blood-forming tissues of the bone marrow go berserk, reproducing at an uncontrolled rate and sabo- taging the function of normal blood cells. The cancer cells deprive the body of much-needed oxygen and rob it of the ability to fight infection. As the disease

Lindsay Conner

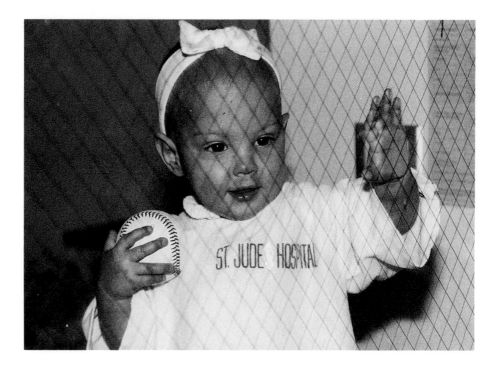

progresses, the cancer cells move throughout the body, invading vital organs through the blood stream. Acute leukemias progress rapidly and if untreated are fatal within a few months. Early detection is crucial in combatting this disease.

When Lindsay was diagnosed with AML, her doctor referred her to St. Jude Children's Research Hospital, and Lindsay's parents put their daughter in the car and drove to Memphis from their Heyworth, Illinois, home. "At first when we got here, I didn't trust anybody," says Stan about his initial impression of the hospital. The couple was in a strange place in a distant city with the frightening knowledge that their child might die. They thought they might never be able to take Lindsay back home.

When Lindsay was admitted, she became one of the more than 4,800 children listed as active patients at St. Jude that year. An active patient is a child who is participating in a research protocol to study his or her illness. In 1994, about 43 percent of St. Jude's patients were enrolled in a protocol for one of the forms of leukemia; about 48.9 percent were being followed by the solid tumor service; 4.5 percent were enrolled in hematological studies; and 3.6 percent were in infectious disease or immunology studies.

A few months later, Lindsay's parents had reason for hope. Lindsay achieved remission in October 1992, after chemotherapy treatments and an autologous bone marrow transplant using her own bone marrow. A bone marrow test in February 1993 showed no trace of cancer cells.

"She's a fighter," says Susan proudly. Lindsay's nature, sensitive and resilient, helped her cope with the separation from her sister and the side effects of her chemotherapy. Kept apart from the people she loved by a hospital room window during her treatments, Lindsay remained the charming little girl she had always been. That tough spirit and the care she received at St. Jude made the difference.

"Now that we've been here, I'd be afraid to take her anywhere else," says Stan. "There's never been a day they've done something to Lindsay without telling us first, explaining it to us, and you just start to trust everybody the nursing staff, the doctors, everybody."

Successful treatment of pediatric leukemias, more than anything else, put St. Jude Children's Research Hospital on the medical map. Always striving for a cure, researchers stretched the limits of medical knowledge of pediatric leukemias, adopting such novel approaches as irradiating the brain and spine and injecting anti-leukemic drugs directly into the spinal fluid in order to destroy leukemic cells in the central nervous system — the most common site of relapse. Today such therapies mean that at least 96 percent of children with ALL enter remission after intensive multi-drug treatment.

While achieving remission is an important milestone in the treatment of leukemia, it by no means indicates the end of therapy. Leukemia is treated with chemotherapy, and sometimes radiation therapy, for approximately two to three years. Initial therapy to induce remission for ALL normally requires four to eight weeks of hospitalization or continual daily visits to the hospital. Normally, after a child reaches remission, he or she returns home for what St. Jude calls continuation therapy. At this point, the child commutes to the hospital for periodic clinic visits, but also receives treatments and checkups by a family doctor who uses a treatment method designed by St. Jude physicians. These family doctors work closely with the hospital staff, following St. Jude's research plan and administering expensive drugs supplied by the hospital. St. Jude's five affiliates also provide continuation therapy services for St. Jude patients in their facilities, using the treatment program designed by the child's St. Jude doctor. St. Jude Children's Research Hospital is the primary care provider for all its patients. Even if the child is receiving care from an affiliate or a local physician, he or she always returns to St. Jude at various intervals for examination and treatment as required.

Through St. Jude Children's Research Hospital's treatment methods, cure has become a reality for childhood leukemia victims. Overall, more than 70 percent of St. Jude's ALL patients are cured, and those with the more common standard-risk ALL have a better than 80 percent chance of survival.

Unfortunately, AML has proven to be a more onerous adversary, due to its resistance to all but a handful of drugs. Even in the most successful U.S. studies, children with AML have had no more than a 40 percent chance of being cured by chemotherapy alone. This depressing statistic has spurred searches for novel types of anti-cancer drugs that might eradicate the resistant leukemic cells that cause patients to relapse. One of the most promising candidates is known as 2-CDA. The medicine was synthesized and first tested at St. Jude and in relapsed patients has proven effective.

In order to fight Lindsay's battle with AML, doctors at St. Jude performed a bone marrow transplant. Bone marrow transplants offer hope to leukemia patients who don't respond to chemotherapy and radiation. The two types of bone marrow transplants — allogeneic, in which bone marrow cells from a related or unrelated donor are infused into the patient's circulatory system, and autologous, in which a small amount of the patient's own marrow is removed and purged of cancerous cells, then reinfused — have had widely varying success rates, from 10 percent to 70 or 80 percent. Researchers are now investigating the field of genetics for clues to enhance the chances of a successful outcome for bone marrow transplants and answer questions about the origins of childhood leukemia.

Looking always in the direction of increased survival rates, St. Jude researchers anticipate the day that children diagnosed with AML will face better odds. It is hoped that advances in drug therapy and bone marrow transplants may some day bring AML survival rates to the encouraging level of standard risk ALL.

Debbie and Mark Mask will never forget the day in May 1992 when their six-month-old son, Taylor, became ill. Debbie had gone shopping, leaving Mark and Taylor at home, when the boy started vomiting and his eyes rolled back in his head. Alarmed, Mark called and left messages at all the stores he knew his wife would visit. When Debbie got the message, she rushed home to see about her son. One look and she knew that Taylor was very sick, so the couple rushed Taylor to a children's hospital in Memphis. By the time they arrived there from their Southaven, Mississippi, home, Taylor was unresponsive. "He was breathing, but he was limp," Debbie remembers.

A CAT scan of Taylor's skull revealed a tumor the size of a baseball on the lining of his brain. Known as a choroid plexus carcinoma, the tumor was a rare form of childhood cancer. Taylor was admitted to the hospital's intensive

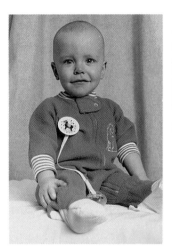

(Left) Taylor Mask

(Right) Emily Kahn

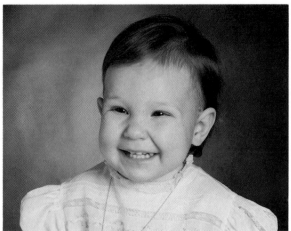

care unit, where nine hours later he stopped breathing. A ventilator was hooked up to keep him alive. When his condition had stabilized somewhat a few days later, he underwent eight hours of surgery to remove the tumor. By that time, it had permanently destroyed the sight in Taylor's right eye.

Taylor's doctor referred him to St. Jude Children's Research Hospital. Two weeks after his admittance, he began chemotherapy. After 11 of 16 scheduled treatments, Taylor's doctor at St. Jude decided to take Taylor off treatment, since the drugs were beginning to affect his hearing.

From the very beginning, Debbie and Mark were counseled that if Taylor's tumor came back, he would have little chance of long-term survival. But more than a year and a half later, Taylor's periodic checkups at St. Jude still looked good. The feisty little boy was slowed down by his fight with cancer, but only temporarily. "It took Taylor about six months to get back on track," Debbie says.

Brain tumors are the second most common childhood cancer after leukemia, representing 20 percent of all pediatric malignancies. Each year in the United States approximately 1,500 new cases of brain cancer are diagnosed in children under the age of 15. In 1984, St. Jude researchers began researching and treating the more than 30 identified types of brain tumors.

Unfortunately, brain cancer has proven to be a formidable enemy. The average success rate for treatment of brain tumors in children is about 45%. For children under 2 years of age, long-term survival has not exceeded 20 to 30 percent, disheartening statistics since one in eight brain tumors occur in infants and young children under the age of 2.

The problem is multifaceted, but one roadblock has been the diversity in types and treatment responses. Because differing responses among the many types of brain tumors have inhibited the collection of information on any one type, programs of research and treatment specifically for children with brain tumors have been slow to develop. The real hope for the future is both in more effective treatment and earlier tumor detection. Further research may indicate what causes brain tumors and what features are indicative of malignant behavior, critical information for understanding these tumors and developing critically needed new treatment strategies.

Treatment for brain tumors includes surgery, radiation therapy and chemotherapy, with surgery almost always the first step. At St. Jude, radiation therapy is delayed as long as possible to avoid any possible long-term effects on the brain, particularly in children under the age of 3, whose brain cells are still developing and are particularly sensitive to high energy X-rays. The traditional order of performing surgery first, followed by radiation therapy and sometimes chemotherapy, has changed in an attempt to use chemotherapy when it may be the most effective: immediately after surgery and prior to radiation. Researchers expect that this will also help reduce learning problems in children who now have a chance for survival.

Selected tumors that are unreachable with conventional surgery may be treated with stereotactic radiation, a procedure that uses carefully focused beams of X-radiation to shrink the tumor without harming other areas of the brain. Brachytherapy is also being investigated as a treatment for brain tumors. In brachytherapy, radioactive seeds — pellets of radioactive iodine — contained in plastic tubes are implanted around the tumor. Each tube remains in place about four days. This treatment provides high doses of radiation to the tumor without toxic side effects to healthy tissue nearby.

St. Jude Children's Research Hospital has made a commitment to increasing the odds for children with brain cancer. In so doing, more lucky children will be around to see their next birthday, like little Taylor Mask.

Before dawn one morning in October 1993, 4-month-old Emily Kahn awakened her parents, Randa and Stanley, with her crying. Emily was normally a contented baby, but that morning nothing would console her. As the hours passed and nothing seemed to comfort her daughter, Randa decided Emily must be suffering from an ear infection and she would call her doctor as soon as his office opened. At 8 a.m., Emily went limp; by 8:30 her eyes started to cross. Frantic, Randa called her pediatrician and said she was bringing Emily in. After seeing the child, the pediatrician could not calm Randa's fears. When asked if Emily was going to be all right, he could only say, "I can't tell you that right now."

Immediately, Randa rushed her daughter to a local hospital for tests. "The tumor was actually pressing on her pancreas," she explains, "and at that time, she was having a hypoglycemic seizure. As soon as they got the right fluids going, she was fine, at least for that day."

Emily was diagnosed with neuroblastoma, the second most common childhood solid tumor after brain tumors. The tumor was pressing on Emily's diaphragm, liver and kidney, and an operation to remove it was successful. Also removed was one of Emily's adrenal glands and a cancerous lymph node.

The cancer diagnosis was a complete shock to the Kahns. Emily had seemed so normal since birth. In retrospect, Randa is thankful that her child experienced the seizure that October morning. "Looking back on it now, I'm glad it happened," she says, "because if it hadn't happened that way, we'd never have known, and the tumor would have kept growing."

Emily's doctor referred the family to St. Jude, and Dr. Laura Bowman, an expert in the treatment of children with neuroblastoma, took over Emily's care. Dr. Bowman told the Kahns that Emily's chances for long-term survival looked good.

Neuroblastoma is a complex solid tumor arising in cells that form the sympathetic nervous system. Found only in children, this solid tumor develops from primitive nerves cells growing abnormally. More than 50 percent of cases of neuroblastoma occur in the adrenal glands in the abdominal area near the kidney.

Neuroblastoma presents unusual challenges to pediatric oncologists. Children whose tumors are localized are likely to be cured with standard treatments. Once the tumor has spread, however, the outcome depends on the child's age and on specific genetic features of the tumor cells. Bone marrow transplants are used for children over 1 year of age whose tumors have spread, but with localized tumors, surgery is sufficient almost 100 percent of the time.

Emily's chemotherapy treatments ended in February 1994, and a second surgery to determine if there were any problems had good results. After her follow-up surgery, Emily was scheduled to return to St. Jude every three months for checkups. "To me, St. Jude and Dr. Bowman gave me my daughter back," says Randa, "because without them I wouldn't have her here today."

St. Jude's work in neuroblastoma is seen as one of the hospital's most important medical achievements. In 1962, the survival rate for neuroblastoma was only around 10 percent. In 1976, Dr. Alexander A. Green and Dr. F. Ann Hayes developed treatment techniques that doubled the length of remission for the disease, giving them more time to treat patients. At the time, this was considered to be a major breakthrough because it allowed different approaches to be used which in turn led to increased survival rates. Today, improved intensive chemotherapy has increased overall four-year survival rates to 55 percent; for infants with neuroblastoma, the survival rates have increased to about 89 percent. Any child stricken with neuroblastoma can now expect a significantly increased chance of survival if treated on protocols similar to those developed by St. Jude research physicians.

Scott Hinshelwood was a freshman in high school when his left ankle began to hurt. Since Scott was an avid basketball player, he thought the pain was probably due to a sprain. "It wasn't excruciating, but when I landed on it a certain way, the pain shot up my leg," Scott says. The next month, May 1990, Scott went to see a doctor friend of the family. When the doctor took X-rays of the leg, Scott's osteosarcoma was exposed.

Osteosarcoma, a fast-spreading malignant tumor of the bone and the most common form of bone cancer in children, occurs most often in bones on either side of the knee or in the upper arm. Usually seen in children and young people between the ages of 10 and 25, it is more frequently found in males. It is usually treated by amputation of the affected limb, followed by chemotherapy to prevent the spread of malignant cells to other parts of the body. St. Jude has achieved a 60 percent survival rate for osteosarcoma, up from 15 percent 30 years ago.

When Scott's doctor recommended that he go to St. Jude Children's Research Hospital, Scott was stunned. He had come to the doctor thinking he had some minor ailment. "I was kind of excited about wearing a cast and to be on crutches and have people feeling sorry for me." A referral to St. Jude was the last thing he had expected.

The week after he was admitted, Scott started his course of chemotherapy treatments, and within two weeks, his hair had completely fallen out. Unfortunately, the drugs failed to shrink Scott's tumor.

The tumor was growing into his foot rather than up his leg, which was an advantage, since as Scott explains, "If it had gone upward, I probably would have lost my leg higher up." As it was, a month after Scott's diagnosis, his leg was amputated right below the knee.

After the surgery, Scott says, "I had a lot of phantom pain where your brain thinks your foot's there and sends signals. Your toes will burn and itch, and it hurts like crazy, because it feels like somebody's stabbing your foot."

Today some patients faced with the loss of a limb can often avoid the trauma of amputation by opting for limb-salvage surgery, which consists of

(Left) Scott Hinshelwood

(Right) Katie Cyran

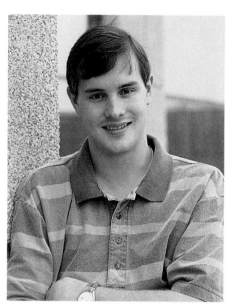 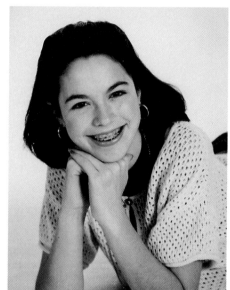

removing the involved bone and surrounding tissue while preserving the neuromuscular bundle. About three-fourths of osteosarcoma patients are eligible for this procedure; however, some choose to have the amputation rather than the reconstructive surgery, since jogging and contact sports are impossible after the limb-salvage surgery.

Scott's chemotherapy treatments ended in March 1991. After that, he began a series of follow up checkups at the hospital. "I lost a little quickness in basketball, and I can't jump as high, but I can still do everything I did before I lost my leg," he says about his condition.

Through it all, Scott never lost his wry sense of humor. In a discussion about his pending amputation, Scott turned to his surgeon and said, "I want it back." The surgeon looked at his young patient blankly and said, "Son, you don't want your leg back." "It's my leg isn't it?" Scott replied. "I want to mount it and put it on my fireplace."

When Katie Cyran was 6 years old, her doctor advised her to stay out of gym class. She had been experiencing pain in her chest, and her physician thought she might have pulled a muscle. Katie didn't appear to be sick during the day, but at night the pain would escalate, and her abstinence from physical activity didn't alleviate her discomfort.

Finally, after several months went by without lasting relief, Katie's doctor ordered some tests. A scan revealed a growth the size of an orange on one of Katie's left ribs. It was Ewing sarcoma, a solid tumor affecting the bone shaft.

Ewing sarcoma, the second most common type of bone cancer, is frequently found in the flat bones, such as the pelvis, as well as the proximal bones of the extremities, the upper tibia and ribs. It oftentimes spreads to other bones and the lungs. In the early 1960s, Ewing sarcoma was 95 percent fatal. In 1995, the overall survival rate climbed to 60 percent. For patients with a localized tumor, long-term disease-free survival is about 70 percent. Those with metastatic tumors at diagnosis fare worse; but even 30 to 50 percent of these patients can enjoy long-term survival and potential cure.

Katie's parents, Linda and Frank Cyran, were very familiar with St. Jude Children's Research Hospital when Katie's doctor recommended that she become a patient there. They had sent regular donations to the hospital and quickly agreed that it would be the best place for their daughter.

After Katie was admitted, she was given six months of chemotherapy, and on July 3, 1986, her tumor was surgically removed, along with her sixth rib and some of her seventh. "They thought the tumor would be completely dead," Linda says, "but the center was still alive." Surgery was followed by six weeks of radiation therapy and more anti-cancer drugs.

Katie's intense therapy was very rigorous for the little girl. She was sick most of the time and lost a tremendous amount of weight. Nonetheless, at the end of her treatments, her physician at St. Jude said she had an 80 percent chance of being cured.

By the time Katie was 14, she was enrolled in St. Jude's After Completion of Therapy (ACT) Clinic for patients who are off treatment and doing well. She still runs the risk of developing a secondary cancer because of the radiation, but fortunately has shown no adverse signs.

When Katie was first diagnosed with cancer, her parents immediately prayed to St. Jude. Their faith and their daughter's fortitude and courage pulled Katie through a devastating ordeal — that, and the research and care available at St. Jude's Children's Research Hospital.

Carolina Martinez was a very frightened child when she came to the United States. The 9-year-old adopted daughter of Luis and Pablina Martinez had been diagnosed with a malignant lump on her nose at a hospital in Santiago, Chile. She lay sobbing in a hospital bed there, her wrists tied down to keep her from ripping out the intravenous line in her arm, as her parents desperately searched for a way to keep their daughter alive. The couple had two other adopted children, and they could never afford to pay for the expensive cancer treatments that Carolina needed.

Carolina Martinez and parents

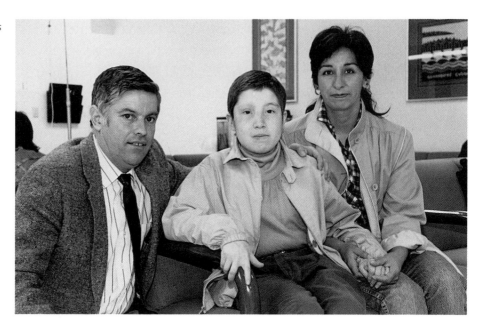

Fortunately, Carolina's doctor thought of St. Jude Children's Research Hospital. After her physician telephoned the hospital and described Carolina's condition, she was accepted for treatment. On April 28, 1992, Carolina was admitted to the hospital as a patient. Angelica Acchiardo, a fellow Chilean who works at St. Jude as an international volunteer and translator, was waiting for Carolina when she arrived.

"I was here when she first came, and it was terrible," Angelica recalls. "She was so scared from her experiences in the hospital in Chile...she cried every time someone came into the room."

Carolina's treatments for rhabdomyosarcoma, a childhood cancer arising in muscle cells, consisted of chemotherapy and nine weeks of radiation. Proper diagnosis of sarcomas is crucial, but the tiny size of the structures makes their distinction very difficult. Fortunately, the last 10 years have brought the development of powerful tools to aid in their identification, making diagnosis faster and more reliable.

Also crucial in Carolina's case was the concern shown for her by the doctors and nurses who treated her. "She got confidence," says Angelica, "when she saw that the people at St. Jude Hospital had so much love for her and were so nice to her."

Fortunately, the combination of therapies worked for Carolina, and after a year in the United States, she and her parents returned to their home in Chile, where Carolina was scheduled to have regular checkups. Because of the medical care Carolina received at St. Jude, she can now look forward to a promising future. A little girl who cried at the sight of strangers left St. Jude giving hugs to the friends she had made there.

When Todd McKinley returned home one day in the late summer of 1986, his parents were waiting for him. The teenager had noticed "knots" on his neck shortly before and had shown them to his mother, Linda. She felt the lumps and, somewhat surprised by their hardness, urged her son to stop in at a minor emergency clinic for a checkup. The tentative diagnosis was mononucleosis.

Todd's follow up visit at his regular doctor revealed something more. An X-ray showed a suspicious looking shadow, or mass, and the family's surgeon performed a biopsy.

The phone call from their surgeon after the results were known was what prompted Bill and Linda McKinley to sit in their home dreading their son's arrival. The surgeon had informed the McKinleys that Todd had cancer. "That's the hardest thing I ever had to tell him, that he had cancer," Linda says about that day. Stunned, all Todd could say was, "Can I be cured?"

Todd was diagnosed with Hodgkin disease, cancer of the lymphatic system. His doctor referred him to St. Jude Children's Research Hospital. When the family arrived there, they sat, holding hands, in their car. The McKinleys, like so many families before them, looked to God for support. "Lord," Linda prayed, "we don't know what's behind those doors or what to expect, but we just leave it all up to you."

The cancers known as lymphomas account for about 10 percent of childhood cancers. Lymphomas are divided into Hodgkin disease and non-Hodgkin lymphoma. Non-Hodgkin lymphoma commonly affects the abdominal organs but can also appear in the neck, chest or elsewhere. The cure rate at St. Jude for non-Hodgkin lymphoma is 80 percent, up from its former 6 percent, making it one of the most curable forms of childhood cancer if detected in the early stages.

Hodgkin disease involves the lymph nodes, especially those in the neck. It may spread to the liver, spleen, bone marrow and lungs. Once considered uniformly fatal, Hodgkin disease is now 90 percent curable in its early stages through the use of a chemotherapy and radiation combination therapy developed, in large part, at St. Jude.

Because of his treatments, Todd's appetite disappeared, and he lost weight. "They were always on me about eating," he recalls. "When I found out I had Hodgkin disease, I weighed about 135 pounds, but after my treatments, I was down to about 112 pounds." Fortunately, Todd's disease was in a relatively

Todd McKinley with his wife and daughter

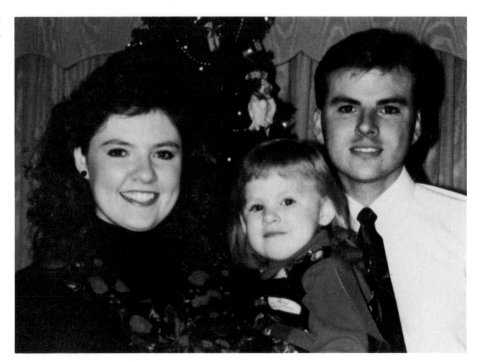

early stage, and his course of radiation treatments was successful. He remembers that the treatments made him tired, but quickly adds, "I remember how supportive the nurses were at St. Jude Hospital — they went out of their way".

Todd is considered cured. He still returns to the hospital for yearly checkups, but cancer is now a part of his past. His life today includes a wife and two children, and the knowledge that St. Jude was one of the reasons that this life is possible.

Todd, Carolina, Katie, Lindsay, Taylor, Emily and Scott are only a very few of the many children who have put their lives in the hands of St. Jude. Their diseases only represent a sampling of the illnesses researched and treated in the hospital's laboratories and clinics. Fortunately, in the case of most catastrophic childhood diseases studied at St. Jude, increased survival rates attest to significant progress in the battle against childhood cancers and other illnesses.

For many childhood cancer patients, however, infection poses as serious a threat to their survival as did their primary disease. Radiation and chemotherapy weaken a patient's resistance to normal childhood illnesses and retard the ability to recover when infected. Moreover, the hospital setting exposes children with cancer to organisms about which little is known.

For this reason, one of the most crucial areas of research at St. Jude is infectious diseases. This department investigates infections occurring in children with defective host defenses. These include bacteria, viruses and fungi that rarely, if ever, cause serious infections in otherwise healthy children, but may produce life-threatening complications in patients receiving cancer therapy.

In 1977, Dr. Walter T. Hughes, chairman of St. Jude's infectious diseases division, developed the first preventative therapy for one of the most dangerous threats to cancer patients: *Pneumocystis carinii* pneumonia (PCP). A stock drug — trimethoprim-sulfamethoxazole (TMP-SMZ) — was found to be almost 100 percent effective against PCP in patients with compromised immune systems. Since that time, TMP-SMZ has become a standard part of treatment for patients in danger of developing PCP.

PCP also claims the lives of victims of pediatric AIDS. Thus in tandem with treating and protecting cancer patients from infectious diseases, doctors and scientists at St. Jude are conducting intensive research studies to combat infectious diseases for patients with pediatric AIDS.

Even though AIDS was not a disease that people wanted to talk about, Danny Thomas felt it had to be addressed, which he did during the groundbreaking ceremony for the start of the 1987 expansion program. At a major news conference following the ceremony, Danny and Dr. Hughes announced the hospital's initial enrollment of children with AIDS. Today, St. Jude Children's Research Hospital is one of 22 research centers that make up the AIDS Clinical Trials Unit, which is supported by the National Institutes of Health. St. Jude's infectious diseases division houses the pediatric AIDS program, aimed at helping those whom Thomas referred to as AIDS' "most innocent victims."

In 1994, the World Health Organization estimated that 1,500,000 infants worldwide have contracted HIV since the start of the pandemic. In the United States, more than 4,000 children younger than 13 are infected with the disease. Unlike pediatric cancers, which through the years have had a fairly steady rate of occurrence, AIDS is on the rise, especially among adolescents. Currently, no patient can be cured of AIDS. Drug therapy merely prolongs life for a few years on average.

In infants, the incubation period for the HIV virus is much shorter than in adults, with symptoms of infection appearing by about three or four months of age. "They have a more rapid downhill course," says Dr. Hughes.

Since almost all children with pediatric AIDS contracted the disease from their mother, the progress made at St. Jude in its efforts to prevent transmission of the virus from an HIV-infected mother to her unborn child is encouraging. St. Jude played a large role in a national study that showed that the drug AZT decreased the risk of transmission of the HIV virus to the unborn children of pregnant HIV-positive women by about two-thirds. This study was the first evidence that pediatric AIDS can be prevented, and should have a dramatic impact in reducing the number of pediatric AIDS cases every year.

In addition to investigating *Pneumocystis carinii* pneumonia in pediatric AIDS, the hospital's scientists are researching new drugs for other opportunistic infections that occur in AIDS patients, such as cryptosporidiosis, an intestinal and pulmonary disease. The consensus among scientists seems to be that it is unlikely that drugs will be found soon that will actually cure AIDS. Yet anti-viral drug combinations targeting specific steps in the viral cycle will undoubtedly prove indispensable, both in treating the opportunistic infections that are the hallmark of AIDS and in combating the actual infection.

"I think we have to assume that in the next five to 10 years, all the therapeutics are going to treat AIDS as a chronic disease," says Dr. Arnold Fridland, an associate member in infectious diseases. "AIDS will still be a fatal disease, but people will be living longer with the infection."

St. Jude is also studying HIV on the molecular level. A vaccine would be one way of generating the incredible diversity that an AIDS vaccine would need. Hundreds of different types of viruses could be presented in a DNA-type vaccine. However, DNA vaccines are years away because their safety and efficacy is not yet proven.

Dr. Randy Owens, an assistant member in virology and molecular biology, believes, "If you look at HIV research with a historical perspective, I think you will see that research on AIDS has gone considerably faster than that of most other viruses. A vaccine is going to be difficult to produce, much more difficult than an influenza vaccine, for instance. But I wouldn't be working on it, and I don't think anybody else here would be working as hard as they are either, if we didn't think it could be done."

Unlike the study of pediatric AIDS, which began at St. Jude in the late 1980s, the search for a cure for sickle cell disease has been a part of St. Jude Children's Research Hospital since its beginnings, thanks to the influence of Dr. Lemuel Diggs, a pioneer in the study of the disease.

Sickle cell disease is a genetic disease primarily of African-Americans and affects one of every 350 black newborns in the United States. It also affects people from Asian, Central American and Mediterranean origins. In sickle cell disease patients, normal, pliable, doughnut-shaped red blood cells become rigid and sickle-shaped. The distorted cells cannot pass easily through small blood vessels, which results in problems such as severe pain, life-threatening infection, organ damage and stroke.

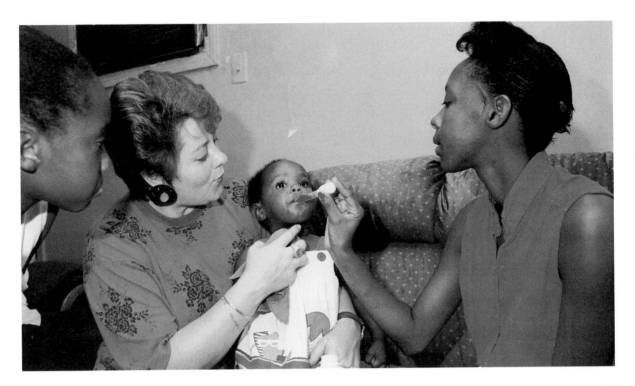

A home visit is made for a sickle cell disease patient.

At present, there is no cure for sickle cell disease, so treatment is aimed at preventing and treating complications. Bloodstream infection has been the leading killer of young sickle cell disease patients, but aggressive preventive efforts and more effective antibiotics have resulted in more sickle cell disease patients being able to receive treatment on an outpatient basis when they are seen for infection-induced fevers.

Research at St. Jude indicates that bone marrow transplants using the marrow from genetically matched donors may eradicate sickle cell permanently. The first bone marrow transplant for a patient with sickle cell disease was performed at St. Jude in 1982. The donor's marrow was transplanted to treat his brother's leukemia, but it also unexpectedly cured the child's sickle cell disease.

However, given the risks of donor transplants and the scarcity of matched donors, this treatment is best viewed as a stepping stone toward improved therapies. The ideal therapy would be applicable to all patients and would not carry the toxicity associated with bone marrow transplantation. Toward that end, St. Jude is focusing on sickle cell gene therapy, which may provide the ultimate treatment, introducing corrected genes into the patient, genes that will then produce the normal red blood cell. protein, hemoglobin.

Sickle cell disease, pediatric AIDS, brain tumors, high-risk leukemias — these are some of the challenges still facing the physicians and scientists at St. Jude Children's Research Hospital. As they look increasingly toward new avenues for research and treatment, there is always the hope that the next protocol, the next clinical trial, or the next laboratory experiment will open a door to the better understanding of pediatric diseases and how they can best be treated, prevented and cured.

Their mission so far has been marked by tremendous success, as more and more patients return home disease-free to recommence their lives and parents put their sons and daughters to bed at night without wondering if that day was their last. Nonetheless, St. Jude Children's Research Hospital and ALSAC are accelerating their efforts, rather than slowing down, and have dedicated themselves to continuing their work as long as there are catastrophic diseases of childhood. For no matter the illness, Danny believed, and frequently used, an old Arabic adage, "No child should die in the dawn of life."

WE ARE A FAMILY

You will never know how much you are doing for all the mothers. I can't believe there are so many good people in this world. I still have a son because of you.

Patricia Miranda, mother of St. Jude patient Marko Miranda

The doctors — Dr. Santana, Dr. Mirro — are superb, and the rest of the staff are wonderful.

Gayle Williams, commenting on St. Jude.
Her daughter, Heather, was lost to AML in 1989
after a long battle, including a bone marrow transplant.

The most beautiful aspect of this facility is the great outpouring of love and affection from the entire staff.

Lucy Shober, mother of Wren Shober
who lost her battle with leukemia
on January 15, 1990, at the age of 3

It should not be surprising that in spite of the tremendous advances St. Jude Children's Research Hospital has made against catastrophic childhood diseases, some children still die. Consider that even though overall survival rates for acute lymphocytic leukemia, the most common form of childhood cancer, are now 73 percent instead of the 5 percent rate of 1962, odds are that three of 10 children will not make it. What is surprising to those just learning about the hospital is the love that parents, even those who lose a child there, have for St. Jude. They, better than most, know how necessary it is for research at St. Jude to continue. There are good reasons for this unusual devotion. They are found in the care and concern received not just from the medical staff but shown by everyone from top to bottom, from volunteers as well as employees.

St. Jude Children's Research Hospital never closes its doors to the small victims of childhood's catastrophic diseases. Newly diagnosed patients arrive at the hospital at all times of day and night. Since more than half of the patients live more than 200 miles from the hospital, many must face an unfamiliar environment in city far from home. Afraid to even contemplate the future, families come and place their trust in St. Jude. From that moment on, the hospital takes over. It will be a part of these young patients existence for the rest of their lives.

Mothers and fathers of St. Jude's patients confront crises no parent should ever have to face. However, one major area of concern for many parents of other stricken children does not affect St. Jude families. Because of the financial support of ALSAC, St. Jude Children's Research Hospital parents have never had to pay for any part of their child's treatment. Drugs, radiation therapy, surgery, inpatient care, consultations, follow-up care, even lodging, transportation and meals for the child and one parent are covered by the hospital. Parents who wish to contribute to the cost of treatment are told they can make a donation to ALSAC. ALSAC covers all costs beyond those reimbursed by third party insurers, and all costs when no insurance is available.

The emotional impact of cancer diagnosis and treatment is enormous for everyone involved. Cancer takes a heavy psychological toll on patients, parents and siblings. Nonetheless, since its first patient was admitted, St. Jude Children's Research Hospital has practiced a policy stressing complete honesty in relationships between patient, family and staff. The hospital's first medical

A patient has a birthday party in one of the St. Jude play areas in 1987.

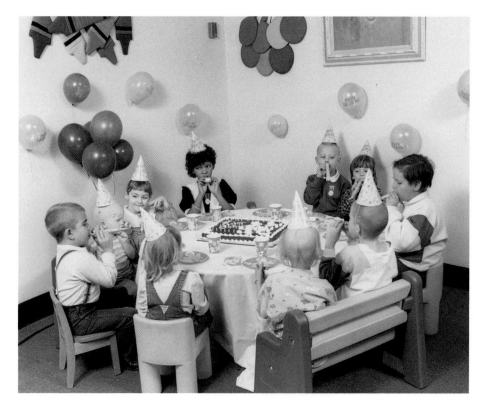

director, Dr. Donald Pinkel, believed that families had a right to know about a child's condition, and that if informed in advance about what was going to happen, they could endure unbelievable stress.

But the family is not left to deal with these stresses on their own. The St. Jude staff perceives the patient and family as one unit, and takes special care to address the needs of everyone affected by the child's diagnosis. A multi-disciplinary team of social workers, psychologists, pastoral counselors and nurses coordinated by the behavioral medicine division offers emotional and practical support to both the patient and family. As one nurse practitioner put it, "We are scientists; we are interested in clinical issues and clinical solutions. But remembering the unique personhood of the family is one of our largest charges and responsibilities. And it is really tremendously satisfying."

Attention to psychological concerns begins when a child is first admitted to the hospital. After an initial physical assessment is completed, a social worker is automatically assigned to the child's case. Based upon the social worker's recommendations, a psycho-social team — composed of the social worker, a psychologist or psychological examiner, a chaplain, a member of the medical or nursing staff, and a child life worker — meet to decide what level of intervention and follow-up the child and family need.

The social worker is primarily concerned with helping the patient and family deal with the stress and turmoil of cancer care. Addressing all needs other than medical, social workers counsel siblings and teachers; help parents with marital strains; assist families in dealing with anger, fear and grief; and serve as a link to community resources. In addition to daily counseling sessions, the social work staff conducts several special workshops for families. Among these are a monthly "Super Sibs" Saturday for patients siblings and a retreat for families coping with a diagnosis of HIV or pediatric AIDS. Hospital chaplains are also available to patients and families seeking spiritual counseling.

Patients who experience acute or chronic adjustment problems related to their illness or treatment can rely on the psychology division for evaluation and consultation. Problems may range from poor compliance with therapy to learning problems in school. Some patients are automatically seen by the psychology department — children with brain tumors, those undergoing bone marrow transplantation, children participating in any of the AIDS Clinical Trials Unit (ACTU) protocols and children with sickle cell disease.

With brain tumor patients, in particular, the department also conducts objective developmental assessments at various stages in treatment to gain an accurate portrayal of the patient's condition. "A longer range goal," says Dr.

St. Jude patient Melinda Swofford, shown with patient Tom Davidson, became a St. Jude nurse following her successful treatment.

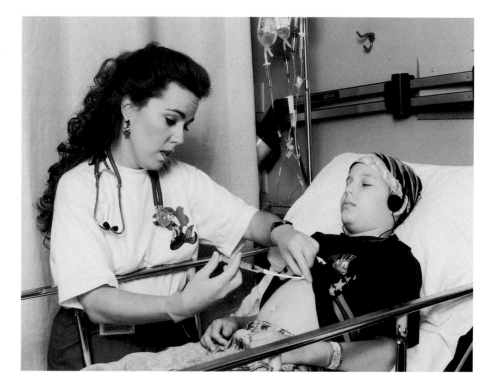

Raymond Mulhern, director of behavioral medicine, "is to be able to eventually identify the amount of toxicity associated with different types of therapy and to be able to report that to the physicians, so that future protocols can be modified to reduce the toxicity." Behavioral medicine's interests lie in defining the impact of therapy on learning and development in order to assess the overall effects of treatment.

In behavioral medicine, psychologists and social workers also conduct studies in such areas as family adjustment to childhood's catastrophic illnesses and special problems experienced by adolescents with malignant diseases requiring amputations. Investigation extends to the study of cancer treatment's long-range psychological ramifications, as well. In the hospital's early years, there was no need to explore long-term effects, since there was no long-term survival. With the ensuing medical advances that pushed survival rates increasingly upward, however, a whole new spectrum of psychological concerns presented itself. Since 1973, when St. Jude Children's Research Hospital's psychiatric program received its first federal grant in the amount of $34,000, attention has been directed at studying such issues as the effects of radiation and long-term treatments and the damage that either might do to the child's learning process and personality long after these treatment are discontinued.

Another major concern at St. Jude is the systematic establishment of as normal and non-threatening an environment as possible for the young patients. The child life program, instituted with the opening of the hospital's Patient Care Center in 1995, is designed to minimize children's stress and anxiety during hospital visits and encourage normalization and development while patients are in the hospital through appropriate play and educational activities. The program works closely with the departments of psychology, social work, nursing and volunteer services.

Each inpatient is assigned a child life worker to spend time with in activities that will promote the child's development. Part of the child life mission is to try to decrease stress associated with hospitalization and help the patient take an active role in his or her treatment.

One technique child life specialists use to clear up misconceptions is medical play. Younger children feel much more secure in unfamiliar situations if they are allowed to talk about and witness medical procedures using dolls. If they can watch a doll being treated, they can get a sense of mastery over what's actually going to be done to them. Child life specialists talk about the fact that it's okay for the doll to cry during an injection, but it's not all right for the doll to move when receiving medicine. By telling the doll what to do, patients learn what their role will be when it's time for them to have the procedure.

In an era in which increasing medical technology and sky-rocketing costs have depersonalized health care, St. Jude Children's Research Hospital has dedicated itself to addressing every aspect of patient and family needs related to treatment. "We want to meet the families' needs beyond just providing medical care for the child," says Dr. William Crist. "We want to treat our families with dignity and convey to them that we're concerned about their quality of life at St. Jude. We want them to know we appreciate their pain and this inconvenience to their lives."

This attention to all aspects of a patient's well-being is one of the hallmarks of St. Jude Children's Research Hospital. It is a complete care concept the hospital pioneered. Along with psychological evaluations and support, the hospital also provides nutrition supplements and counseling; surgery, follow up care and rehabilitation services; and free dental and opthamological care for conditions related to the child's primary illness. This innovative concept was instituted with St. Jude's first leukemia patients. Their treatment involved a combination of chemotherapy and radiation that caused the children to lose all immunity and suffer a variety of side effects. It was necessary for the doctors at St. Jude to have complete control over the child's medical program to effectively treat the primary disease and control the effects of treatment. As a result, no aspect of a child's physical or psychological needs is overlooked when he or she becomes a patient at St. Jude. Dental care is one example.

For a healthy child, dental problems can be severely painful. For a child at St. Jude, they can be life-threatening. Dental infection, like any infection, could kill a child with a weakened immune system. Add to this the fact that chemotherapy and radiotherapy frequently cause oral complications — drying up salivary glands and breaking down teeth — and it becomes clear why dentistry plays an important role in cancer treatment. St. Jude's on-site dental clinic helps provide preventative dental care before beginning treatment or intervention later to avert serious infection, malnutrition and poor response to therapy. The dental clinic also conducts research on the oral and dental effects of cancer and its treatment. Dr. Kenneth Hopkins, a dentist at St. Jude for more than 18 years, has designed a shield to protect patients teeth during irradiation. The clinic has also developed a special rinse to treat mouth ulcers that result from chemotherapy.

Children with chronic, long-term diseases also have special nutritional needs. These needs may increase while food intake decreases, resulting in weight loss and slowed growth. Side effects associated with cancer and cancer treatments may also interfere with normal nutrition processes. Preventing or limiting nutrition problems in the pediatric cancer patient is an important consideration for the St. Jude staff.

Upon admittance, patients are measured and weighed, and a complete diet history is recorded. Registered dieticians monitor patient charts on a continuous basis so that nutrition counseling and intervention measures can be instituted before weight loss becomes a medical problem. The dietician develops a nutrition care plan specially tailored to the patient and his or her treatment, and provides counseling as to what the child should eat at home. Food supplements are provided if the patient is not able to eat enough for a regular diet due to the side effects of treatment, which can include nausea, vomiting, diarrhea and loss of appetite.

Children who are not able to eat may require nutrition through their veins or by a tube inserted directly into their stomachs. A multi-disciplinary team of doctors, nurses, pharmacists, dieticians and social workers is responsible for overseeing the daily care of all patients who require metabolic or nutrition support and providing education to the family on the proper use of equipment, dosages and feeding techniques.

Children with catastrophic diseases also require expert, specialized nursing care. St. Jude Children's Research Hospital's division of nursing encourages excellence and improvement in pediatric oncology skills through constant updates in the intensive care, ambulatory, inpatient and other specialty areas. In addition, an active nursing research program headed by Dr. Pamela Hinds addresses routine care practices. The larger issues faced by children with life-threatening illnesses, their families and the nurses who provide their care are also studied. Such investigations have included examinations of patients' and parents' coping strategies for dealing with a first recurrence of cancer and identification of the factors considered important to parents, physicians and nurses in their decision-making processes at critical points in treatment.

　　　Since one of the hospital's goals is to provide the best possible quality of life after therapy, everyone is interested in providing care best suited for the whole patient. For the surgery department, that philosophy has manifested itself in the surgery staff's focus on reducing the long-term, as well as acute, effects of surgery using such innovations as modular prostheses and limb salvage. After that comes rehabilitation. But rehabilitation at St. Jude Children's Research Hospital is not considered solely post-operative physical therapy. St. Jude's rehabilitation specialists design activities for maintaining strength, function, endurance and developmental progress throughout the patient's long period of treatment and recovery. Individualized therapeutic or preventive pro-

(Left) Physical therapy session, 1994.

(Right) Nursing assistant Ricky Boatman, also known as the button man, with Bridgette Pemble in 1988.

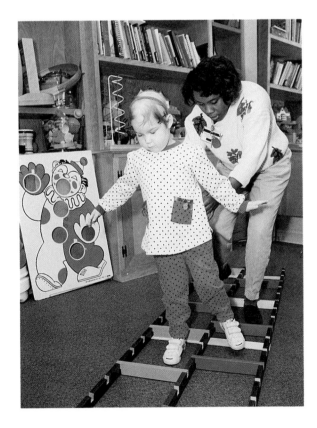

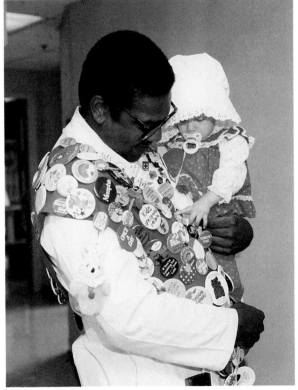

Volunteers help entertain children in several play areas of new patient care center.

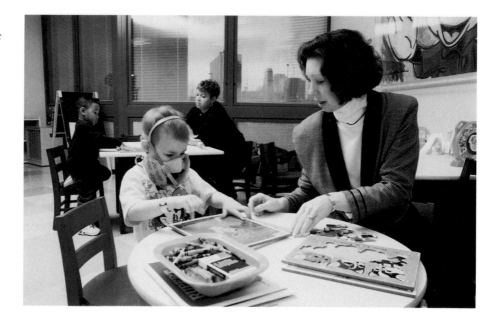

grams combine physical therapy, occupational therapy, speech pathology, audiology and prosthetic and orthotic services tailored to meet the specific needs of each patient.

A candidate for bone marrow transplant, for example, visits a physical therapist before and after surgery. The sessions before the transplant work to build the child's stamina; the postoperative sessions focus on recovery, allowing the child to leave the hospital sooner. Before an amputation, bone tumor patients see physical therapists to work on strengthening the muscles of their unaffected limbs. As a result, most of these patients are up and walking within 24 hours after surgery. They return to normal life quicker and are better equipped to deal with their amputation. Brain tumor patients also gain great benefits from physical therapists, who help them regain and strengthen their balance and motor skills. Occupational therapy and speech therapy also help in their recovery.

Because most rehabilitation work is considered preventive care, therapy is often not covered by insurance. In addition, many insurance policies pay for only one prosthesis during an insured's lifetime. For a 6-year-old child who needs a $10,000 artificial leg every year until he is fully grown, that type of reimbursement will not take him very far.

For this reason, St. Jude's rehabilitation services are truly a "testimony" to its donors. Prosthetics and rehabilitation, like all St. Jude's medical care, are provided to patients without regard to their financial situation. In the case of rehabilitation services, there is little chance that the hospital will receive insurance reimbursements for its expense. St. Jude Children's Research Hospital would be unable to provide this instrumental care if not for the donations received from the public through ALSAC.

Patient care at St. Jude extends long after remission is attained, rehabilitation is complete and a patient returns to everyday life. A patient at St. Jude Children's Research Hospital can usually be considered a patient for life. After completion of their treatment regimens, patients enter a long-term follow up program whose establishment marked a significant milestone in the hospital's history.

Started with more than 1,300 former pediatric cancer patients who had been living disease-free for as long as 20 years, the After Completion of Therapy clinic was intended to meet the challenge of studying the increasing population of childhood cancer survivors. As St. Jude's fastest-growing clinic, ACT focuses on wellness, survival and the future. The clinic's sole purpose is to monitor the survivor population of St. Jude for any residual side effects of cancer therapy and to identify problems that might be corrected in future treatment protocols. Like their colleagues in other clinics, ACT clinic faculty and staff are concerned with every aspect of the patient's health; they want to know about patients educational progress, exact physical status, occurrence of pain and any psychological or social problems they may be dealing with.

Patients are enrolled in the ACT clinic when they reach five years from diagnosis if they have been in continuous remission and have been off all therapy for at least two years. (Enrollment in ACT comes later for those who relapse but have a subsequent continuous remission.) A patient must also be free of any life-threatening diseases. The ACT clinic follows the physical and emotional health of long-term cancer survivors by means of annual physical checkups and psychosocial screening, looking for side effects to treatment and possible problems of acclimating to normal life. Side effects may include growth and development problems, alterations in sexual maturation and reproductive function, or a change in heart, lung, liver, gastrointestinal, kidney or thyroid function.

Dr. Melissa Hudson, a St. Jude oncologist and the clinic's chief, focuses on "quality of life" educational programs to help survivors lead healthy cancer-free lives. Clinic members are taught about their particular type of cancer and cancer therapy and their specific risks for late effects. The clinic staff can often anticipate, prevent and treat conditions that might otherwise cause serious problems. Additionally, the clinic advocates preventative measures to minimize the risk of patients developing a second cancer. Some drugs and radiation treatments can increase the risk of a second (different) cancer. The clinic's staff tells patients how they can lessen this risk and be alert to the early warning signs of cancer.

"The treatment of cancer is neither gentle nor specific," says Debbie Crom, a pediatric nurse practitioner who works in the ACT clinic. "And often long-term survivors are going to have some organ system toxicity. They certainly are going to have life events that reflect the assault upon them early in their life. But those are things often we can intervene into, thus improving their quality of life."

According to Crom, the typical long-term survivor office visit includes blood work, an X-ray, a urinalysis, a careful history and review of systems from top to toe, and a physical examination. After those preliminary events, the ACT staff looks at practical and psychological issues, dealing with the social and emotional side effects that cancer can have. Pediatric hematologists-oncologists, nurse practitioners and RNs work with psychologists and social workers who make up the ACT multi-disciplinary team. Psychological testing, social services and subspecialty referrals are available if needed.

"It still astonishes me in ACT clinic that we have such little 'physiological toxicity,'" says Crom. "These kids are healthy, well and active. But perhaps the greater toxicity they will face is a 'socio-economic' toxicity." Life insurance for cancer survivors is often unavailable. Health insurance coverage is often

(Left) Memphis school teachers help out-of-town patients keep up with school work. Here Susan Pollack helps Monica McCullon with cursive writing lesson in March 1988.

(Right) International volunteers help St. Jude's foreign patients and their families cope with living away from home in a strange land. Maria Chandler at left provides directions for the day to members of her team.

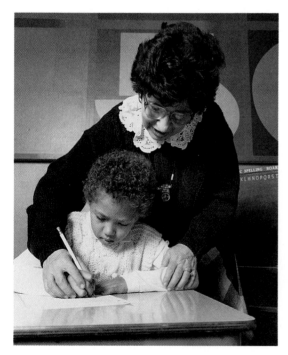

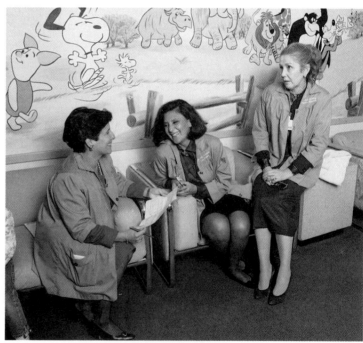

denied for illnesses and circumstances totally unrelated to cancer. Job discrimination against survivors of childhood cancer exists. The hospital, along with other national organizations, has taken on the role of patient advocate in some cases, but it also insists that patients "become people of quality," says Crom, "that have a skill to sell, because they are going to need this in the job market, and they are going to need to be able to rise above it."

Akin to the treatment offered in acute care, this attention to every aspect of the patient's life extends to other members of the family, as well. Many times it is not until the threat of recurrent disease is behind them that family members can begin to voice their feelings and fears. For that reason, the ACT clinic staff wants to support the whole family, educate family members about the specific disease and therapy, and address any questions they may have. Families at home are sent a copy of the patient's physical exam and a list of anticipated problems, as well as assurance about things that will not be problems in the future.

Once enrolled in the ACT clinic, patients are seen once a year until they reach age 18 or are 10 event-free years from their most recent diagnosis, whichever comes later. At that time, they graduate from the ACT clinic and become St. Jude alumni. As of June 1, 1996, there were 1,229 patients in the ACT clinic and 1,202 alumni, for a total of 2,429 survivors of childhood cancer being followed. St. Jude Children's Research Hospital held its 1st Survivor Conference on June 1, 1996, with over 500 former patients, now adults, attending. Although alumni no longer return to St. Jude for yearly visits, the ACT clinic coordinator maintains contact with them through telephone calls and questionnaires, offering assistance in the event that the hospital can be of help should any health problems related to their cancer arise. The ACT team helps prepare patients for alumni status by nurturing their independence through education of the patient and those who come into contact with the patient. Furthermore, the clinic follows patients on a lifetime basis, seeking pertinent research findings for publication as a means of providing information on survivors needs.

While monitoring the health of long-term survivors, the clinic also gathers data about the late effects of therapies. These large-scale studies suggest how treatment protocols can be modified to reduce late toxicities and improve the quality of life for future survivors. "Although the clinic is unique and it is a wonderful opportunity to participate in the lives of our patients, we want to enrich the lives of long-term survivors of childhood cancer everywhere," says Crom. The ACT clinic research agenda addresses six to eight critical items in the lives of long-term survivors of childhood cancers. These include the cardiac integrity of patients after receiving certain drugs, fertility status and quality of life issues such as life satisfaction, self-esteem and physical integrity. Information on side effects influences treatment plans for newly diagnosed patients. Furthermore, appreciation of the late effects of cancer therapy in patients monitored in the clinic has been instrumental in reducing the amounts of chemotherapy and radiation used for treating certain types of cancer.

Before the ACT clinic was established, there was no way of knowing how St. Jude survivors were faring in the mainstream. Today approximately 2,300 patients visit the clinic annually. Says Dr. Hudson, "I think the most important thing for all of us — social work, psychology, the medical team here, the nurses and the doctors — is to try to identify any obstacles to successful survivorship. It may be a physical problem, it may be an emotional problem, it can encompass any aspect of their life, their school performance, their ability to be in a relationship, to make friends, et cetera, so we identify those and try to work with them specifically."

"Intimacy is a lasting commitment to our patients," says Crom. "I think it's been a great commentary on the integrity of our founding fathers and on ALSAC to not desert survivors, to say survival is not enough. We want to do everything we can to improve the quality of life. Not only for the patient that walks in our door today ill for the first time, but also for patients who have been here 10 to 15 years. We are committed to you."

Another outstanding aspect of the treatment at St. Jude is that given by its dedicated volunteers. Putting in countless hours for such simple rewards as a free flu shot or a yearly lunch, these men and women have been a part of St. Jude Children's Research Hospital from its earliest years, even before it opened.

Hospital volunteers gave Ann Brinkmann the idea to come to work at St. Jude. Waiting for treatment one day in the lobby, Ann watched as the volunteers led a group of visitors on a tour. She had been diagnosed with high-risk acute lymphocytic leukemia, so she had ample opportunities to see the volunteers at work. The volunteer who had the strongest impact on Ann appeared one day while she was sitting alone in her hospital room. Her former first grade teacher walked through the door and called her name. "It was wonderful to see that familiar face," Ann remembers. The teacher volunteered regularly on Wednesdays and would always check in to see if Ann was there. "She'd bring me something to cheer me up, something to do, some toys, some stationery, some games, something."

Now working in the volunteer services department, Brinkmann speaks from personal experience when she says, "I think the volunteers really become

Patients Wendy Davis, front, and Lindsey Cook share a happy moment at ALSAC-St. Jude national convention in 1994.

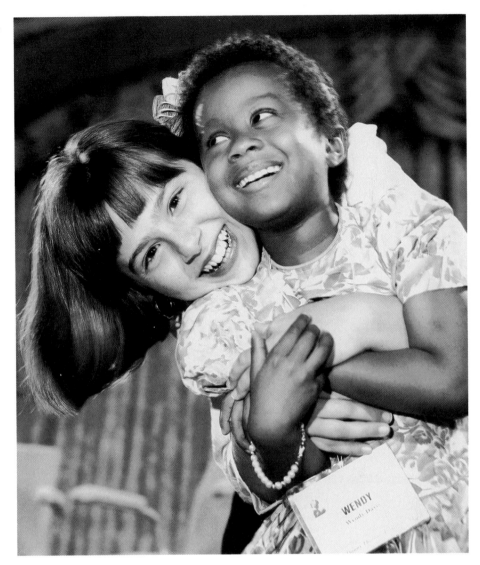

familiar faces for the children. They come here and they are anticipating seeing that volunteer who they are used to playing with. It's like an aunt or uncle to them." According to Ann, the volunteers help keep the patients lives more stable.

Approximately 300 people donate their time and energy as volunteers at St. Jude Children's Research Hospital. Coordinating their efforts is the job of the volunteer services staff, which acts as the liaison between the volunteers and St. Jude Children's Research Hospital departments. Volunteer services recruits, interviews and provides a general orientation for new volunteers, who are then assigned to one of the hospital's departments for more specific training. Denise Gaston, the director of volunteer services, believes the "volunteers are really the glue that holds the hospital together," and have been since Danny Thomas first began spreading the word of his dream. "Danny Thomas knew that the hospital was not going to be able to make it without these volunteers at the very beginning," says Gaston. "Whether it was the ALSAC volunteer gentleman in the business environment going out drumming up funds to get enough money to build the hospital, or whether it was their wives who were helping wash the diapers or get the milk bottles ready or sweep the floors or answering the telephones or handling the paper work. All that was done with volunteers." Three major groups within the hospital now operate under the umbrella of volunteer services: The Ladies of St. Jude, the St. Jude Auxiliary and the St. Jude Women's Club.

Six years before the hospital opened, a group of women — many of whom had close ties to members of Danny Thomas Memphis Steering Committee for St. Jude Hospital, to St. Joseph Hospital or were the wives of Memphis doctors — formed an organization that would soon become the Ladies of St. Jude. Since 1956, when they originally called themselves the St. Jude Auxiliary, these early volunteers have helped the hospital, initially assisting with clerical work and raising funds for the hospital's construction. After the hospital's opening, the Ladies of St. Jude pitched in wherever their help was needed. That meant assisting in the business office, peeling potatoes in the kitchen, scrubbing bathroom floors, working in the pharmacy, raising money to fund a playroom, operating the switchboard, taking patients to appointments at a time when the hospital used many outside doctors, or housing patients during their stays. "There wasn't anything they didn't do to help St. Jude get off the ground," according to Mrs. E. Bradley Clasgens, long time member and archivist of the Ladies of St. Jude.

The earliest members of the Ladies of St. Jude when it was formed included Mrs. James Dillion (the first president), Mrs. Emmet Werne, Mrs. Charles C. Drennon (Catherine), Mrs. Robert Lawrence, Mrs. William D. Baldwin (Elizabeth), Mrs. Nat Buring (Sylvia), Mrs. Frank Tobey (Lucille). Mrs. John T. Dwyer (Leona) and Mrs. Clara Marmann joined in 1960. The name was changed to Ladies of St. Jude that year. One of the early members of the group was Helen Hogan, who served as a volunteer in the pharmacy, writing letters to pharmaceutical houses requesting complimentary drugs, before she was recruited by Dr. Pinkel to work for him as a volunteer for two years. Later she was hired full time at St. Jude and worked for more than 20 years as secretary for Dr. Allan Granoff.

Today the Ladies of St. Jude is primarily a fund-raising organization committed to raising money for specific needs not covered in the hospital's regular budget. The organization has provided the hospital with such generous contributions as bone marrow transplant equipment, infant ventilators, a bloodmobile, leukemia parent/patient educational booklets, chapel supplies and copy machines.

"People who enjoy working with children, who want to help St. Jude Hospital and who have a genuine interest in seeing children in a hospitalized setting feel better" are the kinds of people who volunteer at St. Jude, says Gaston.

The St. Jude Auxiliary (no relation to the original 1956 St. Jude Auxiliary), the largest of the hospital's volunteer groups, is made up of women and men representing every type of background from all walks of life. The Auxiliary has programs geared for teens, college students, internationals and anyone else who wants to make a commitment to helping the children of St. Jude. St. Jude Auxiliary volunteers work with patients in the hospital's recreation areas as well as helping in the research labs, offices and the gift shop. They also give tours to hospital visitors.

With the opening of the Patient Care Center, Gaston has seen new playrooms provide additional recreational space for the children in settings specifically geared for different age groups. That additional space and the institution of the new child life program at St. Jude, focusing on the growth and development of the hospitalized child, have increased the possibilities for volunteer interaction with the children.

Volunteers like Jenny Bledsoe, a retired school teacher who runs the patient library and has been coming to St. Jude Children's Research Hospital to help out for more than a decade, play vital roles in both the St. Jude Auxiliary and the lives of St. Jude's young patients. Outpatients can depend on volunteers to be in their play areas offering instruction, entertainment and support. In addition, a "toy lady" visits the inpatient rooms each morning to see what each child wants to play with that day. Volunteers visit with the children for 30 minutes to an hour, playing games and helping with homework, and, in addition, giving the parents a much-needed break.

Evolving out of St. Jude's successful Hispanic Volunteer Program of the 1980s, today's International Volunteer Program is organized to meet the needs of St. Jude's increasingly diverse foreign patient population. As Mrs. Lottie Richards, Voluntarios Hispanicos member in 1985 said, "We're happy to help families from Spanish-speaking countries who receive treatment at St. Jude. It shows what a beautiful job the hospital does in caring for all the children around the world." Now that assistance is extended to families from Europe, Asia and Africa, as well.

Jeanne Dycus, social work director and the Hispanic Volunteer Program coordinator in the early 1980s, says, "These families need much more help than American patients. For most it means a move for the entire family, because treatment can extend from a few months to two-and-a-half years." Social workers assist the families with initial arrangements, then the hospital's international volunteers provide crucial help in such necessary activities as finding housing, enrolling siblings in schools, locating language courses and establishing bank accounts.

The international volunteers, many of whom were born in a foreign land themselves, also serve as translators for foreign patients and their parents. They come from Europe, Asia, and Latin America and are an important part of the St. Jude Auxiliary. They are probably the most intensely trained of all St. Jude's volunteers. According to international volunteer Maria Chandler, who coordinated the program's expansion, the program is "designed to help families maintain their identity and reinforce their culture, something we feel can be better accomplished through group activities involving all international patients." The volunteers, who undergo six weeks of training from the social work department, are fluent in translating medical terms and providing information in a compassionate, understanding manner. They provide immeasurable support to families who not only are coping with the shock and fear of having a gravely ill child but are also in an unfamiliar culture far from home.

The St. Jude Women's Club comprises another of St. Jude's invaluable groups of volunteers. Composed of female hospital faculty and the wives of St. Jude male faculty and staff, the members of this group help families of employees new to the Memphis area. Serving as a welcoming committee, the St. Jude Women's Club assists new arrivals with everything from investigating the local housing market to locating stores to furnish new homes. The Women's Club is also in charge of decorating the hospital during the holiday season, providing more than 40 trees to brighten the patients' surroundings.

"Our total focus every day is how we can make the patients more comfortable and how we can make it a happier, more cheerful place and make their experience less traumatic, says Gaston. This concern for the patients' well-being extends to all members of the family. "We really focus on the patients, the siblings and the families as a unit. Whenever we say the patient, we really mean the brothers and sisters and the parents, because everybody is involved."

In its role as a goodwill messenger for the hospital, volunteer services also serves as the toy depository for the hospital. Toys donated to St. Jude are stored in its offices, always available for a child who is celebrating a birthday or the end of treatment, or who just needs a little something special to make the day seem a bit brighter.

Although they are not paid for their time and efforts, the St. Jude Children's Research Hospital volunteers find rewards that mean much more. Lorraine Willis, one of three volunteers who visits the parents' rooms on the inpatient floors each morning, remembers one 12-year-old boy who was having a difficult time coping with the recent amputation of his leg and refused to get out of bed. Concerned, his nurse told the "Toy Lady" about him. Willis suggested that they hang a basketball hoop over his bathroom door, saying, "Don't ask him to throw, because he'll resist you. Just throw one in." The nurse threw the ball as the boy watched. Sure enough, climbing out of the bed, the boy said, "I can beat you." A St. Jude doctor once said to Willis, "I treat them. You make them happy."

Quo Vadis?

The way you people talk you'd think I did this whole thing myself with a pen knife and shovel.

Danny Thomas, 1987

I get tired sometimes but every time I think I'm going to quit I visit St. Jude...

Danny Thomas, 1980

On February 6, 1991, Danny Thomas died of a massive heart attack at the age of 79.

"Danny Thomas was not a figurehead in our fund-raising," said Baddia J. Rashid, ALSAC's national executive director at the time of Thomas' death. "Even up until today, Danny was our leader, and he personally participated in as many events as he could. In all these years of leadership, Danny not only contributed several million dollars of his own money, but he became the catalyst that brought millions of donors and volunteers to the support of his dream."

St. Jude Children's Research Hospital was Danny Thomas' pride. He was the founder, leader and patriarch of St. Jude Hospital as well as its chief fund-raiser for nearly 40 years. No mere celebrity condescending to lend his name to a worthy cause, Danny Thomas venerated St. Jude and honored his promise to the saint to the end.

"I get tired sometimes," Thomas remarked 10 years before his death, "and every time I think I'm going to quit, I visit St. Jude. And going through the hospital and seeing those kids, especially the ones who aren't going to make it, I just go out and rededicate myself. I really just want to go out in to the street and mug somebody for his money if he won't give it to me."

A man of lesser caliber would have been satisfied with Danny's phenomenal success in Hollywood as a TV star and producer. Danny won five Emmy Awards for his television show *Make Room for Daddy*, and was a partner in the production of such hits as *The Andy Griffith Show, The Dick Van Dyke Show, The Real McCoys* and *The Mod Squad*. Nonetheless, Thomas always used his

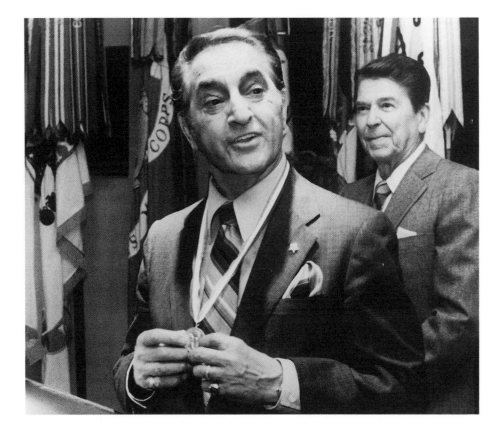

success to further the cause of ALSAC and St. Jude Children's Research Hospital rather than supplant it.

"Dad's impact on television and show business was tremendous," says his daughter Terre Thomas. He was the picture of decency and he was in real life the way he was on TV — dynamic and loving." He was responsible for many great and wholesome TV shows being on the air. While known by the public primarily for his work in front of the camera, Danny Thomas and his partner Sheldon Leonard were in reality among the industry's pioneer producers and developers of new talent.

Danny was a frequent visitor to the hospital — a man who always walked in the front door, greeting all the children in the lobby, a man who talked to the children, comforted them, held them and tried to brighten their days with a loving presence and gentle humor.

Two days before his death, Danny came to Memphis to film a fundraising commercial, and while there he and Rose Marie joined patients, parents and employees in celebrating the hospital's 29th anniversary on February 4, 1991— the first time they had been in Memphis on that date since the hospital's opening in 1962. His autobiography, *Make Room for Danny*, had just been published, and a book signing was held in the rotunda of the Danny Thomas/ALSAC Pavilion. During that visit, Thomas ironically pointed over his shoulder toward the mausoleum and said, "I just want to live as long as the Lord allows and then come here to be buried."

These prophetic words were among his last wishes. After services in California and Memphis, Thomas was laid to rest in a family crypt at the pavilion on the grounds of the hospital. While Danny lay in state at the pavilion, lines of patients and their families and thousands of Memphians passed by his casket to pay their respects to the Thomas family and to a man of vision and extraordinary compassion. White roses are placed at his crypt daily by his family as a reminder to visitors, families of patients and the thousands of children who benefitted from his caring that Danny Thomas' dream will live on.

"I believe show business has only been a vehicle to fulfill my destiny to establish St. Jude," Danny Thomas once remarked. "Founding that hospital is the highlight of my life. Thousands of children are alive today who otherwise would be dead if that place wasn't there.

"We see the kids that survived from 1962 to 1967, and they are not kids any more. They're adults and living a good life, some with children of their own. If we'd done nothing more than that, it would have been worth it."

In a statement issued at the time of Thomas' death, then-medical director Dr. Joseph V. Simone reflected, "Our response to this tragedy will be to redouble our efforts to save children and to respond to a more recent charge by Danny to endow St. Jude in perpetuity. We should all be so fortunate when we depart this life to leave such a thriving, humane legacy to the world."

Danny's spirit will always be a part of ALSAC and St. Jude. The bronze bust of Thomas located in the hospital lobby is a constant reminder of his devo-

(Left) Danny's last live visit to St. Jude was on Monday, Feb. 4, 1991. He came to Memphis to tape a set of new fund-raising commercials. It was the first time since 1962 that he had been in Memphis on the anniversary of the hospital's dedication. With Rose Marie, Dr. Joseph V. Simone and ALSAC-St. Jude's national executive secretary Sandra Vogel Lewis, he helped celebrate the hospital's 29th anniversary at a ceremony in the hospital's cafeteria.

(Right) Danny's last official act at St. Jude Children's Research Hospital was to autograph copies of his new book, Make Room For Danny, in the ALSAC-Danny Thomas Pavilion. During that appearance in the evening Feb. 4, he told several people that he would be buried in the crypt of the pavilion. He flew home to Los Angeles late that evening and died of a massive heart attack shortly after midnight on Wednesday, Feb. 6, 1991. He was 79.

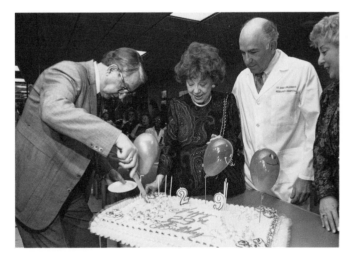

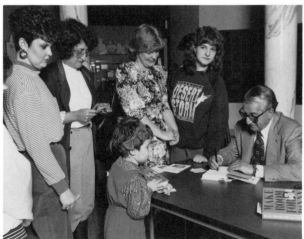

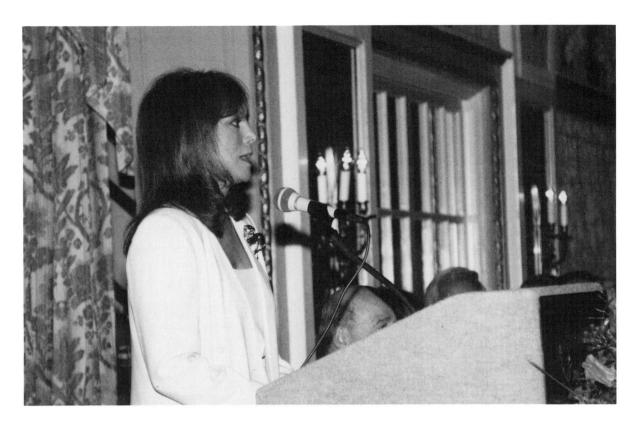

Danny's children continue his work. Here Marlo gives the kick-off speech for a $250 million endowment campaign in 1991.

tion to helping sick children regardless of their race, creed or economic status. The statue has been rubbed to a dull sheen by the hands of young patients, who still stroke the nose as a good luck charm before their treatment. Today, members of the Thomas family — Danny's wife, Rose Marie, and their children, Marlo, Terre and Tony — are totally committed to helping ALSAC and St. Jude fulfill Danny's dream that no child suffer a tragic death from an incurable disease.

Marlo says, "Every visit to St. Jude Children's Research Hospital reminds me of how much my father loved the children here, and somehow I know he's still pulling for them."

She remembers an incident from her childhood that she feels explains in part Danny's commitment to St. Jude. "When I was a little girl, I was driving with my father when we passed a group of boys who were beating up on another little boy. He stopped the car, jumped out, pulled them apart and gave them a talking to. When he got back in the car, he said he hated a bully. I think my father saw cancer in children as a bully. And that's why he worked so hard to build St. Jude Children's Research Hospital. I think he wanted to rescue children from the greatest bully of all."

Son Tony says, "St. Jude Children's Research Hospital has been part of my life as long as I can remember. It is a miraculous institution that is saving thousands of children's lives. For me not to help its pioneering work would be soulless, and it would be denying my father's existence." Terre Thomas has served on the ALSAC-St. Jude board since 1980, and together with Marlo and Tony, they have stepped in to fill the void left by Danny's death. "It is impossible for anyone to take our father's place," Terre says, "and it is taking all three of us, but we mean to see that the dream lives on."

Time has begun to enhance his stature, but to those who knew him and loved him, Danny Thomas will always be the humble man who loved the bologna sandwiches and country fried eggs he fixed for himself in the hospital kitchen, the man who preferred to travel alone with Inspector Dave Wing of the Shelby Country Sheriff's Department in an unmarked squad car, never a limousine, the man who disliked pomposity of any sort and pricked it wherever he found it. Danny never forgot his heritage or the fact that he owed his fame to ordinary people. He was as much at home in the parlor of a blue collar home as he was in corporate board rooms. Perhaps that is one of the secrets of his success in raising money for St. Jude Children's Research Hospital, as much as it was in his success as an entertainer. He realized that it was on the strength of millions of donors giving what they could that gave St. Jude the funds needed for its life-saving work.

Danny Thomas' spirit, charisma and recognition of roots continues as ALSAC-St. Jude Children's Research Hospital prepares to move into the 21st century.

On fund-raising directions, Anthony Shaker, chairman of the board of ALSAC, says, "We must actively try not to stem, but to accommodate reasonable growth. We are looking at growth in television, radiothons, golf tournaments and are testing new programs all the time. We try to adjust to what people like. If they enjoy golf, we want to combine that with our fund raising. We want to make it a pleasure for them to give." Shaker sees planned giving, corporate gifts and other major gift areas as offering the best opportunities for increased revenue.

Like the Thomas family, Shaker has a strong faith in the legacy of Danny and his followers. "Our fathers motives were pure. They were to help sick children, to honor their forefathers, and to thank the United States for liberty and the economic success they achieved. It is essential that these motives stay unchanged. We intend to keep our motives pure."

Although Danny did not live to see the hospital expansion he started in 1987 completed, he would have approved of the decisions the board has taken in recent years regarding the direction of St. Jude Children's Research Hospital,

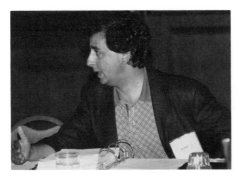 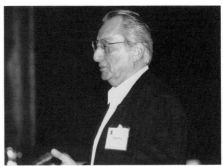

(Left) Anthony Shaker, son of founding board member Joseph R. Shaker, is now chairman of the board of ALSAC.

(Right) Camille Sarrouf, chairman of the board of St. Jude Children s Research Hospital.

in particular those somewhat expanding the admission criteria. St. Jude medical director Dr. Arthur Nienhuis says, "The policy of accepting only newly diagnosed, previously untreated patients is being reconsidered because there is now a need for promising but untested new therapeutic approaches. The hospital opened with the dedication to provide care for children whose illness seemed hopeless. Thus, commitment of a portion of our resources to care for children with advanced disease and poor prognosis is entirely consistent with the hospital's mission."

Camille Sarrouf, chairman of the board of St. Jude Children's Research Hospital, emphasizes that the board is dedicated to providing the best care for all patients. "We are committed to our mission to provide the highest quality of medical care and to develop protocols of treatment that will one day lead to the eradication of catastrophic childhood diseases. Now we plan on taking better care of those admitted from foreign countries. While these patients are restricted to a limited number of our high priority research protocols and constitute a very small part of our patient load, we intend to provide them with the best of care and treatment while they are in America." This extends the long-standing policy of assisting families beyond their immediate medical needs and relieving the financial burden of their stay in Memphis to families from other countries.

Recent developments show the continuing leadership of St. Jude Children's Research Hospital in the world of biomedical science. In 1995, Dr. Peter Doherty, holder of the Michael F. Tamer Endowed Chair For Immunology Biomedical Research at St. Jude, won the Lasker Basic Research Award, following in the footsteps of Dr. Donald Pinkel, who received this prestigious award in 1972; Dr. Charles Sherr was elected to the National Academy of Sciences; Dr. Larry Kun was elected as a Fellow in the American College of Radiology,; William Evans, Pharm. D., was awarded a second consecutive NIH MERIT grant, and Dr. Tom Look received the Award for Excellence in Research from the American Academy of Pediatrics.

New directions in research such as Dr. Amar Gajjar's work in gene transfer therapy, which could provide hope in fighting brain tumors, are being developed today, just as innovative and somewhat radical in their own right as were the hospital's Total Therapy Protocols for ALL in 1962.

The miracle of St. Jude Children's Research Hospital outlined in the preceding chapters continues to thrive in the spirit and attitude of those who give it their loyal support. Anthony Shaker expects growth in other areas as well. "I see continued use of affiliates, which of necessity must include clinics in other centers. We want to expand board membership to other parts of the United States where there is no representation at present. The board is 100 percent behind reasonable growth."

Pointing to the hospital today as the result of the dedication of those who rallied to Danny's call in 1957, ALSAC's current national executive director, Richard C. Shadyac says, "I want the American public to understand that if this small group of people could accomplish this, it can be done over and over and over again. If people are willing to undertake commitments and follow through, dreams can be realized.

"But you'll never ever make it reality unless you dream, and that's what Danny did."

Dr. Michael Debakey once said, "One child saved at St. Jude Children's Research Hospital means one thousand saved elsewhere." That statement dramatically expresses the hospital's mission for the children of the world, as each day and each year sees the vow made by Danny Thomas so many years ago thrive and continue.

St. Jude Children's Research Hospital is an institution that has given and will continue to give to the medical world far more than Danny Thomas even remotely thought of when he prayed to St. Jude Thaddeus in 1940. Yet from his promise came a dream, and from that dream came the reality of St. Jude Children's Research Hospital, a living memorial to one of the greatest humanitarians of the 20th century, Mr. Danny Thomas.

A Year for Brian

reflections by Brian's mother, Sallie Needham

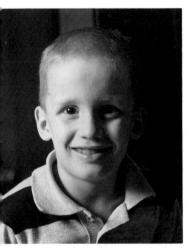

Brian Needham

Was it just a year ago, we were living the life of the average American family? Three kids: Amie, Tim, and three-year-old Brian. Ted and I could handle most of their crises with some encouragement here, a hug and a kiss there.

Then we found that hard, knobby spot on Brian's leg. And we realized he was favoring that leg — swinging it out when he walked.

We didn't panic, but we went to see the doctor. "A cyst," he said, but he sent us to an orthopedic surgeon to be sure. Then the ugly truth emerged. A tumor. Malignant.

Brian had Ewing sarcoma — a bone cancer. But in Brian's case, the cancer was out of the bone. It was, however, dangerously close to the artery.

They removed what they could from Brian's leg, but the battle was just beginning. "Take him to St. Jude Hospital," the doctors said. . . .

St. Jude was not your ordinary hospital. The hubbub in the lobby. All those kids — some playing, some crying, some still and quiet.

It's overwhelming at first, but one thing stands out in my memory. As long as I live, I'll never forget the other parents we met those first few days. The words of reassurance and advice, the warm hand clasps, the comforting smiles. God bless them all.

Brian's St. Jude doctor, Dr. Thompson, soon had Brian on chemotherapy. The treatments are difficult. Brian copes with sickness and losing all his hair. But at least he can be at home, playing with Amie and Tim when he's up to it.

It hurt Ted and me to watch Brian get quieter, paler as he fought the nausea from his treatments. Our bright, bouncy boy who loves to climb trees, so sick.

October — Brian's fourth birthday. Candles, cake, "Happy Birthday to You." His thin face lit by the glow of the candles. How many more birthdays for him?

That day in November at St. Jude. Another tumor. The cancer was back. The fight to get Brian into remission intensifies.

Thanksgiving day — Thank you Lord, for giving us Brian. For his laughter, his love, his quick mind. Thank you for St. Jude, and the way they've helped Brian. Thank you for the people who give to St. Jude to keep the hospital going for the kids like Brian.

Early December — A blow to our hearts. Brian's left leg has to be amputated. How our hearts ache for him. He is so brave, and all we can do is be there for him. And pray. Pray that our precious son will live. There are so many trees left to climb, Brian.

Christmas — Brian's cancer couldn't rob us of the Christmas season's magic, but it added a different perspective. We live one day at a time, happy to be together. Funny how something like cancer gives life such a focus. We're so much more aware of every moment.

I've really grown to love the people at St. Jude. What would we do without them? Their understanding and compassion. The way they take the burden off our shoulders, take care of all the fussy little details when we're there. . .meals, hotel reservations, transportation. We can concentrate on Brian.

I used to know St. Jude simply as the place that Danny Thomas talks about. I hate to think where we'd be — where Brian would be — without St. Jude.

It's strange to think there are people I've never met who have made such a difference in my son's life. People who give to keep this hospital open. People who made sure it opened in the first place. I wish I could thank each one personally.

Spring is coming again. Flowers, green leaves on the trees, birds and the fresh smell of earth.

We keep praying for a cure. We know one thing: Brian has a chance, thanks to the dedicated people at St. Jude.

There will always be a special place in our hearts for St. Jude. St. Jude has given us the most priceless gift — hope for Brian's future.

Brian Needham died of Ewing sarcoma in July 1988, three months short of his fifth birthday. St. Jude Children's Research Hospital and American Lebanese Syrian Associated Charities are committed to working toward that day when children like Brian will be able to climb all the trees they can find.

BOARD OF GOVERNORS AND DIRECTORS

BOARD OF GOVERNORS AND DIRECTORS

1957 To Present

This list includes all who have served as voting members of the American Lebanese Syrian Associated Charities and St. Jude Children's Research Hospital national boards. The Board of Directors of ALSAC and the Board of Governors of St. Jude Children's Research Hospital are legally separate corporations. Their boards consist of volunteer members who serve without compensation to provide the oversight and general guidance to the professional staffs of the two organizations. As explained in the text of this book, there were differences in the membership of the boards when the two organizations were incorporated, but since 1972 the same individuals have comprised both boards. Officer titles for the St. Jude Children s Research Hospital Board of Governors have remained the same since incorporation, but those of theALSAC Board of Directors have changed. To avoid confusion in regard to the relative ranking of offices held, the old titles have been converted to the currently used titles for the same position. Since records from the earliest years are incomplete, this listing has been reconstructed from the best data available. Any omission or error, particularly in listing the officer positions held, is purely unintentional.

Ralph Abercia ....1991 - present

Senator James Abourezk ....1973 - 1976

Alex Aboussie ....1961 - 1968
First Vice-Chairman, Board of Directors — 1962 - 1964

Edward Aboussie ....1967 - 1969

Joyce Aboussie ....1983 - present

Louis Aboussie...1962 - 1965

Anthony Abraham ....1958 - present
First Vice-Chairman, Board of Directors — 1960- 1962

Thomas Abraham ....1988 - present

Moris Adland, M.D. ....1973 - 1978

Susan Aguillard, M.D...1994 - present

Alice Albert ....1980 - 1988

Michael Alcorn ....1986 - 1987

Sister Alfreda, O.S.F. ....1960 - 1962

Nasser Al Rashid ....1987 - 1988

Johnnie Dacus Amonette ....1995 - present

Robert S. Andrews...1960 - 1962

George D. Attea ....1962 - 1969, 1973 - 1975

Mitchell Awn ....1966 - 1969

Joseph A. Ayoub ....1957 - 1974

Joseph S. Ayoub, Jr. ....1989 - present

Joseph S. Ayoub ....1957 - present

Paul J. Ayoub ....1992 - present

Edward F. Barry ....1960 - 1983
    Chairman, Board of Governors — 1960 - 1982
    Chairman Emeritus — 1982 - 1983

Naef K. Basile, M.D. ....1957 - 1978
    Second Vice-Chairman, Board of Directors, 1957 - 1959

Jack A. Belz ....1985 - present

Sister M. Bernardine, O.S.F. ....1963 - 1968

Michael Berry ....1974 - 1979

Elizabeth Beshara..1968 - 1980

James M. Beshara...1981 - 1984

Martha Beshears ....1991 - 1992

William F. Bitar ....1959 - 1963

William Boonisar...1970 - 1977

Michael Borane ....1962 - 1963

John Bourisk, Sr...1960 - 1994

John Bourisk, Jr. ....1992 - present

Thomas Boutrous, M.D ....1957 - 1967

Nat Buring ....1963 - 1976

Ben Cammarata ....1994 - 1995

Barbara Campbell...1995 - 1996

V. Reo Campian ....1967 - present

John Ford Canale...1960 - 1982
  Secretary, Board of Governors — 1962 - 1992

Phyllis Cash ....1990 - 1991

Elias J. Chalhub ....1957 - 1975

DeEtta Charpie...1987 - 1988

Anthony Colonna...1978 - 1987

Sam Cooper ....1974 - 1979, 1985 - present
  Second Vice Chairman, Board of Governors — 1979
  Second Vice-Chairman, Board of Directors — 1976 - 1978

Dr. Joseph Cory ....1992 - present

George Coury..1975 - 1979

George P. Dakmak ....1958 - 1965
  Second Vice-Chairman, Board of Directors — 1964 - 1966

Leslie Dale ....1984 - present

Edward Mike Davis 1970

S. Robert Davis ....1970 - 1971

Robby Dawkins ....1989 - 1990

Peter G. Decker, Jr. ....1971 - 1976, 1978 - present
    Chairman, Board of Directors — 1984 - 1986
    First Vice-Chairman, Board of Directors — 1982 - 1984
    Second Vice-Chairman, Board of Directors — 1980 - 1982

Richard J. Deeb..1958 - 1963, 1984 - 1985
    Second Vice-President, Board of Directors — 1960 - 1962

Roy J. Deeb ....1962 - 1963

Joseph Demos ....1957 - 1970

L. W. Diggs, M.D...1960 - 1975

Lewis R. Donelson ....1986 - present

Patrick Doyle ....1978 - 1987, 1991 - 1992
    First Vice-Chairman, Board of Directors — 1986 - 1987

John T. Dwyer ....1960 - 1965

B. D. Eddie...1957 - 1969
    First Vice-Chairman, Board of Directors — 1957 - 1960

Elias N. Ede ....1982 - 1983

William Edwards ....1957 -
1960

Dr. Edward M. Eissey ....1976 - present
    Chairman, Board of Governors — 1992 - 1994
    Vice-Chairman, Board of Governors — 1990 - 1992
    Secretary, Board of Governors — 1988 - 1990
    Chairman, Board of Directors — 1986 - 1988
    First Vice-Chairman, Board of Directors — 1984 - 1986

Eddie Elias ....1967 - 1972

George Elias, Jr. ....1970 - present
    Chairman, Board of Governors — 1988 - 1990
    Vice-Chairman, Board of Governors — 1986 - 1988
    Secretary, Board of Governors — 1984 - 1986
    Chairman, Board of Directors — 1982 - 1984
    First Vice-Chairman, Board of Directors — 1980 - 1982
    Second Vice-Chairman, Board of Directors — 1979 - 1980

Hasan M. El Khatib ....1985 - present

William F. Farha...1957 - 1965

Sam Farhat ....1960 - 1985
    Second Vice-Chairman, Board of Directors — 1972 - 1974

Maury Foladare ....1960 - 1994

Mrs. Mitchell Forzley..1957 - 1963

Joan Friend ....1989 - 1990

Mary K. Frost...1992 - 1993

Fred P. Gattas, Sr..1957 - 1992
    Chairman, Board of Governors — 1982 - 1984
    Vice Chairman, Board of Governors — 1962 - 1982
    Secretary, Board of Governors — 1960 - 1962

Fred P. Gattas, Jr. ....1989 - present

Ben Geller ....1965 - 1978

Kay Genovese ....1993 - 1994

Minor George..1957 - 1969

Paul George ....1968 - 1991
    Second Vice-Chairman, Board of Directors — 1984 - 1986

Doris Gosnell...1984 - 1985

Halim G. Habib, M.D. ....1964 - present

Judy Habib..1994 - present

James S. Haboush ....1957 - 1962
    Treasurer, Board of Directors — 1957 - 1962

Bill Haddad ....1973 - 1978

Wade Haddad ....1973 - 1985

Joseph M. Haggar, Jr. ....1962 - 1968, 1983 - present

Emile Hajar ....1962 - 1990
Chairman, Board of Directors — 1970-1972
First Vice-Chairman, Board of Directors — 1968 - 1970
Second Vice-Chairman, Board of Directors — 1966 - 1968

Paul Hajar ....1987 - present
Treasurer, Board of Directors — 1990 - 1992
Second Vice-Chairman, Board of Directors — 1994 - 1996

Sam F. Hamra, Jr. ....1985 - 1991, 1992 - present

Joseph A. Hannan..1992 - present

William Harrington, M.D. ....1975 - 1978

Albert F. Harris..1968 - 1987
Treasurer, Board of Directors — 1986 - 1987

Fred R. Harris...1987 - present

William Hassan, Jr., Ph.D. ....1975 - 1984

Theodore Hazer ....1977 - present
Chairman, Board of Directors — 1990 - 1991
First Vice-Chairman, Board of Directors — 1988 - 1990
Second Vice-Chairman, Board of Directors — 1987 - 1988

Cathy Holsted ....1994 - 1995

Ethel Bekolay Horste ....1960 - present
Treasurer, Board of Directors — 1988 - 1990
Second Vice-Chairman, Board of Directors — 1982 - 1984

Joseph Hyder, Sr. ....1989 - present

Albert Jamail ....1970 - 1985
Treasurer, Board of Directors, 1973 - 1985

Albert Joseph ....1957 - present
Chairman, Board of Governors — 1984 - 1986
Vice-Chairman, Board of Governors — 1982 - 1984
Chairman, Board of Directors — 1978 - 1980
First Vice-Chairman, Board of Directors — 1976 - 1978

George Joseph ....1961 - 1962
Chairman, Board of Directors — 1960 - 1962
Second Vice-Chairman, Board of Directors — 1959

Mike McKool 1963

Howard Metzenbaum ....1974 - 1976

Tony Michaels ....1970 - 1975

Fred Mickel ....1963 - 1981

Dr. Corinne Milburn ....1986 - 1987

Ed S. Miller ....1971 - 1976

John P. Moses ....1989 - present
First Vice-Chairman, Board of Directors — 1994 - 1996
Second Vice-Chairman, Board of Directors — 1992 - 1994

Grace Mullenix ....1984 - 1985

James Naifeh ....1985 - present

Richard Naify ....1974 - 1980

Victor Najjar, M.D ....1968 - 1984

George Najour ....1968 - 1969

Floyd Nassif, M.D..1964 - 1975

David B. Nimer ....1984 - present
Treasurer, Board of Directors — 1992 - 1994

Talat M. Othman ....1990 - present

Edward J. Peters ....1968 - 1971

Tom Quick...1991 - present
Treasurer, Board of Directors — 1994 - 1996

Baddia J. Rashid ....1959 - 1976, 1992 - present**
Chairman, Board of Directors — 1962 - 1964
First Vice-Chairman, Board of Directors — 1974 - 1976

Joseph G. Rashid ....1957 - 1968
Chairman, Board of Directors — 1957 - 1959

LaVonne Rashid ....1957 - 1974
National Executive Secretary — 1957 - 1974*

Edward W. Reed, M.D ....1978 - present
Secretary, Board of Governors — 1986 - 1988, 1990 - 1996

Emile Reggie ....1957 - 1977, 1981 - present
First Vice-Chairman, Board of Directors — 1972 - 1974
Second Vice-Chairman, Board of Directors — 1970 - 1972

Fred J. Reggie ....1992 - present

Joseph Robbie ....1961 - 1979
Chairman, Board of Directors — 1966 - 1968
First Vice-Chairman, Board of Directors — 1964 - 1966

Tim Robbie ....1991 - 1994

J. Richard Rossie ....1980 - 1982

Louis Saad, Sr. ....1966 - 1977

George Sabbag ....1972 - present
Chairman, Board of Directors — 1976 - 1978
Second Vice-Chairman, Board of Directors — 1974 - 1976

John Sakakini ....1957 - 1960

Robert T. Salem ....1968 - 1973

Sam Salem ....1957 - 1961

Camille F. Sarrouf ....1985 - present
Chairman, Board of Governors — 1994 - 1996
Vice-Chairman, Board of Governors — 1992 - 1994
Chairman, Board of Directors — 1988 - 1990, 1991 - 1992
First Vice-Chairman, Board of Directors — 1987 - 1988

Walter Schlesinger, M.D. ....1968 - 1970

Rita Schroeder ....1962 - 1973

W. W. Scott ....1960 - 1962
   Treasurer, Board of Governors — 1960 - 1962

Richard C. Shadyac ....1963 - 1992
   Chairman, Board of Governors, — 1986 - 1988
   Vice-Chairman, Board of Governors — 1984 - 1986
   Secretary, Board of Governors — 1982 - 1984
   Chairman, Board of Directors — 1964 - 1966, 1974 - 1976

Richard Shadyac, Jr. ....1992 - 1993

Anthony R. Shaker ....1988 - present
   Chairman, Board of Directors — 1994 - 1996
   First Vice-Chairman, Board of Directors — 1992 - 1994
   Second Vice-Chairman, Board of Directors — 1990 - 1992

Joseph G. Shaker ....1991 - present

Joseph R. Shaker ....1975 - present

Alexander Simon, Jr. ....1989 - 1992

George Simon...1962 - present
   Chairman, Board of Directors — 1980 - 1982
   First Vice-Chairman, Board of Directors — 1979 - 1980
   Second Vice-Chairman, Board of Directors — 1978 - 1979

George A. Simon, II ....1991 - present

George R. Simon ....1960 - 1978
   Treasurer, Board of Directors — 1962 - 1972

Paul Simon ....1986 - present
   Chairman, Board of Directors — 1992 - 1994
   First Vice-Chairman, Board of Directors — 1990 - 1992
   Second Vice-Chairman, Board of Directors — 1988 - 1990

Mitchell Sirgany ....1983 - present

George Sissler 1960

Joseph F. Slavik ....1983 - 1994

Frederick W. Smith...1985 - present

Edward D. Soma, M.D..1966 - present
  Vice-Chairman, Board of Governors — 1994 - 1996
  Chairman, Board of Governors — 1990 - 1992
  Vice-Chairman, Board of Governors — 1988 - 1990
  Chairman, Board of Directors — 1968 - 1970
  First Vice-Chairman, Board of Directors — 1966 - 1968

Sister M. Stephanina, O.S.F. ....1960 - 1972

Morris Stoller...1960 - 1986

Victor Swyden ....1958 - 1961
  Chairman, Board of Directors — 1959 - 1960

Michael F. Tamer ....1957 - 1974
  National Executive Director — 1957 - 1974*

Ronald Terry..1986 - present

Adeeb Thomas, D.M.D ....1966 - 1982

Danny Thomas ....1957 - 1991
  President, Board of Directors — 1957 - 1991

John J. Thomas ....1969 - 1991

Marlo Thomas ....1972 - 1975

R. David Thomas ....1978 - 1981, 1995 - present

Rose Marie Thomas ....1991 - present
  President, Board of Directors, 1991 -present

Terre Thomas ....1980 - present

Thomas C. Thomas ....1962 - 1965

Pat Kerr Tigrett...1993 - present

Andy Tobin ....1988 - 1989

Esther Uhelski ....1973 - 1975

Bernie Wagner ....1969 - 1973

Paul H. Wein...1993 - present

Liz White ....1988 - 1989

Rich White ....1975 - 1978

Gary Wilkinson ....1987 - 1988

Robert Woolf ....1975 - 1978

Robert Paul Younes ....1995 - present

Monsour C. Zanaty...1959 - 1961

Paul Ziffren 1960

Ken Zimmerman ....1985 - 1986

*The National Executive Director and National Executive Secretary were officer positions and voting members of the Board until 1974. In 1974 these position were placed in an ex-officio, non-voting status.

**Following his retirement from his position as National Executive Director in 1992, Baddia J. Rashid was re-appointed to the board.

Current Board of Directors and Governors
(as of July 1, 1996)

The same volunteers serve without compensation as the ALSAC Board of Directors and the Board of Governors of St. Jude Children's Research Hospital.

Joseph G. Shaker*
Oak Park, Illinois

Joseph R. Shaker**
Oak Park, Illinois

George A. Simon II
Detroit, Michigan

George Simon Sr.**
Detroit, Michigan

Paul Simon*
Detroit, Michigan

Mitchell Sirgany**
Miami, Florida

Frederick W. Smith
Memphis, Tennessee

Dr. Edward D. Soma*
Silver spring, Maryland

Ronald Terry
Memphis, Tennessee

Mrs. Danny Thomas
Beverly Hills, California

Terre Thomas
Beverly Hills, California

Pat Kerr Tigrett
Memphis, Tennessee

Paul H. Wein
Guilderland, New York

Dr. Robert Younes
Potomac, Maryland

Ex Officio

Dr. Arthur W. Nienhuis
Director
St. Jude Children's Research Hospital
Memphis, Tennessee

Richard Shadyac Sr.
National Executive Director
ALSAC
Falls Church, Virginia

Sandra Vogel Lewis
National Executive Secretary
ALSAC/St. Jude Boards
Memphis, Tennessee

Board Members Emeritus

In 1989, the Board of Directors
and Governors created an honorary
body to recognize distinguished
service on the Board by those
unable to provide continued active
participation. Members Emeritus
are entitled to all other privileges
of board Members and may participate as they are able, but cannot
vote.

Officers of the Boards

ALSAC

Rose Marie Thomas
President

Anthony R. Shaker
Chairman

John P. Moses
First Vice-Chairman

Paul Hajar
Second Vice-Chairman

Tom Quick
Treasurer

SJCRH

Camille F. Sarrouf
Chairman

Edward D. Soma. M.D.
Vice-Chairman

Dr. Edward W. Reed
Secretary

**Scientific Advisory Board
November 1995**

O. Michael Colvin, M.D.
Director, Duke Comprehensive
    Cancer Center
Duke University Medical Center
Durham, NC

Y. W. Kan, M.D.
Louis K. Diamond
Professor of Hematology,
University of CA, San Francisco
San Francisco, CA

John H. Kersey, M.D.
University of Minnesota
Minneapolis, MN

I. George Miller, M.D.
Professor and Section Chief
Dept. of Pediatrics & Infectious
    Diseases
Yale University School of Medicine
New Haven, CT

Stephen E. Sallan, M.D.
Chief of Staff
Dana-Farber Cancer Institute
Boston, MA

Larry J. Shapiro, M.D.
Professor and Chair
Department of Pediatrics
University of California,
    San Francisco
School of Medicine
San Francisco, CA

Owen Witte, M.D.
Howard Hughes Medical Inst.
University of California
Los Angeles, CA

*   Member,Executive Management
    Board
** Emeritus

ALSAC Offices

Note: ALSAC staff and regional offices provide information, guidance and assistance to volunteers, donors and the general public on fund raising matters. Names and addresses are subject to change, however, as new programs develop or geographical shifts are made. If you are unable to contact any of the offices listed below, please call the National Executive Office for assistance.

ALSAC National Executive Office
P.O. Box 3704
501 St. Jude Place
Memphis, TN 38105
1-800-877-5833

Regional Offices

Northeast Region (1)
505 Eighth Ave., Suite 2210
New York, NY 10018
1-800-526-9542

Associate Office (Region 1)
Three Edgewater Drive, Suite 201
Norwood, MA 02062
1-800-341-5800

Mid-Atlantic Region (2)
6521 Arlington Blvd., Suite 500
Falls Church, VA 22042
1-800-336-3083

Southeast Region (3)
3000 Langford Road, Unit 600
Norcross, GA   30071
1-800-654-8563

Associate Office (Region 3)
401 W. Linton Blvd.
Suite 201
Delray Beach, FL 33444
1-800/278-3383

Central Region (4)
215 W. Muhammad Ali Blvd.
Louisville, KY 40202
1-800 545-1696

Southern Region (5)
2175 Business Center Dr., Suite 7
Memphis, TN 38134
1-800-238-6030

Midwest Region (6)
401 South LaSalle, Suite 1701
Chicago, IL 60605
1-800-621-5359

Southwestern Region (7)
5525 MacArthur Blvd, Suite   500
Irving, TX 75038
1-800-531-5174

Pacific Coast Region (8)
721 S. Parker St., Suite 285
Orange, CA 92668
1-800-227-6737

San Francisco Satellite Office (Region 8)
5994 W. Las Positas Blvd.
Suite 109
Pleasanton, CA 94588
1-800-701-4443

Volunteer Service Centers

Volunteer Service Center I
5796 Shelby Oaks Dr., Suite 6
Memphis, TN 38134
1-800-457-2444

Volunteer Service Center II
510 E. Spring Street
New Albany, IN 47150
1-800-457-2444

Major Gift/Planned Giving Area Offices

Area 10
Three Edgewater Drive, Suite 201
Norwood, MA 02062
1-800-341-5800

Area 11
6521 Arlington Blvd, Suite 500
Falls Church, VA 22042
1-800-336-3083

Area 12
111 Second Ave., NE, Suite 610
St. Petersburg, FL 33701
1-800-648-8905

Area 13
721 S. Parker St., Suite 290
Orange, CA 92668
1-800-894-3592

AFTER WORD

Producing a written history of an institution or organization presents many challenges, foremost of which is selecting and adhering to a cutoff point in time. A history is a snapshot, a picture of what happened up to the deadline when the book must go on the press. Of necessity, everything that happens after the deadline cannot be included nor halt the manufacturing steps that go into printing and production of the book.

The events of October 1996 recall a throw-away line used by Danny Thomas on February 4, 1962, at the opening of the hospital. Just before he pulled the cord to unveil the magnificent statue that stands at the entrance of the hospital, he said, "To those of you who are Catholic, this is a symbol of our faith in St. Jude as the patron saint of hopeless causes and our dedication of this hospital as a shrine fulfilling a promise made to him. To all of you who are of different beliefs, it's still a pretty nice statue."

Danny would have seen St. Jude at work following the announcement on October 7, 1996, that St. Jude Hospital immunologist Dr. Peter Doherty had just been awarded the Nobel Prize for Medicine. He would also have believed that it was not technical problems that allowed this announcement to be inserted in this book after all the proofs had been checked and the first part was actually on the press. He would have said, as he so often did when something wonderful happened at the hospital, that "the fine hand of St. Jude was involved."

Regardless of the cause, the inclusion of the following pages, taken from news releases issued as this book was in the final stages of production, would not have been possible had there not been last minute problems. What would normally have been cause for great concern turned into an opportunity to highlight what is at this time the single greatest tribute to the value and scientific quality of the work of the staff of St. Jude Children's Research Hospital. While Dr. Doherty's honor was for work done before coming to St. Jude, it nonetheless reflects on the high regard in which the hospital is held by the medical and scientific community worldwide. And as Dr. Doherty so readily acknowledges, it was ALSAC and the gifts of millions of its donors that underwrote his work in his first years at St. Jude and has allowed him continue his research along the lines that led to his award. Thus it is truly serendipitous that this After Word section could be added.

If time had permitted, this award would have been incorporated in the text in an uninterrupted flow of the story. As it is, the differences in style and the placement as an addendum are evidence of the last-minute nature of this section. We ask the readers' understanding and forgiveness, and hope that all agree that the significance of the event justifies the form in which it is presented.

As Danny said about the statue, many will simply see this as a stoke of luck for a pretty nice book. But like Danny, many others will add, "Thank you, St. Jude."

Editor, November 3, 1996

St. Jude Children's Research Hospital's First Nobel Prize Laureate

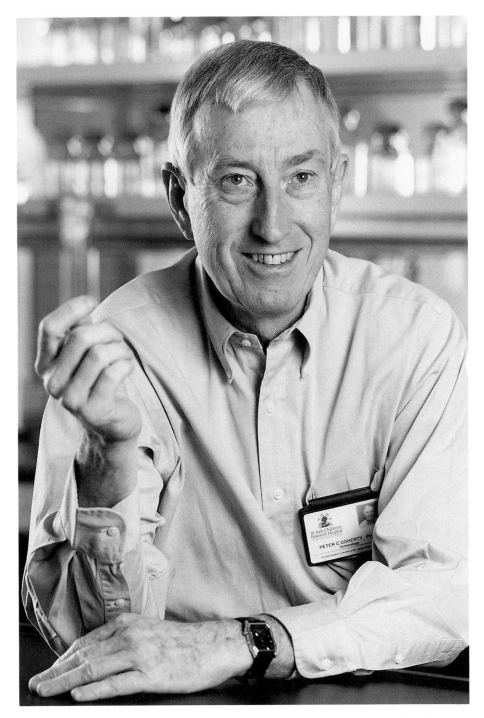

Dr. Peter C. Doherty, Ph.D., chairman of St. Jude Children's Research Hospital's immunology department, was awarded the 1996 Nobel Prize for Medicine.

DR. PETER DOHERTY, ST. JUDE HOSPITAL IMMUNOLOGIST, WINS NOBEL PRIZE

MEMPHIS, October 7, 1996...Peter C. Doherty, Ph.D., and Rolf M. Zinkernagel, M.D., immunologists whose experiments revolutionized the field by explaining the mechanism of T-cell recognition in cell-mediated immunity, have won the 1996 Nobel Prize for Medicine. Dr. Doherty is chairman of the immunology department at St. Jude Children's Research Hospital in Memphis and Dr. Zinkernagel is professor and director of the Institute of Experimental Immunology at the University of Zurich, Switzerland.

Drs. Doherty and Zinkernagel discovered T-cells simultaneously recognize MHC self-protein and a foreign antigen on the surface of virally infected cells. Their discovery of MHS Restriction of T-Cell Recognition opened the door to an understanding of the immune system that has impacted autoimmune disease research, vaccine design, organ transplantation and the understanding of immune surveillance.

Drs. Doherty and Zinkernagel began working together in 1973 at the Australian National University in Canberra. Dr. Doherty joined St. Jude Hospital in 1988.

At a news conference in the ALSAC Danny Thomas Pavilion following the announcement, Dr. Doherty praised the support he received from ALSAC, stating that in 1988 it made his continued research possible.

"I wouldn't be in Memphis without ALSAC. In 1988 I had no grant support and ALSAC provided all my funding until I got my first National Institute of Allergy and Infectious Disease (NIAID) grant. They gave me the Michael F. Tamer Endowed Chair and they still provide a substantial amount of my direct support in addition to underwriting the operation of the entire institution (St. Jude)," Doherty said.

Dr. Doherty's work has had direct impact on advances in the treatment of cancer, AIDS and organ transplant procedures. His award reflects the world class leadership of research at St. Jude.

In September 1995, Drs. Doherty and Zinkernagel received the Albert Lasker Basic Medical Research Award for their work. That award frequently foreshadows the Nobel Prize. Dr. Doherty, also a professor of pediatrics and pathology at the University of Tennessee, Memphis, holds St. Jude Hospital's Michael F. Tamer Endowed Chair for Immunology Biomedical Research. Dr. Doherty is now focusing on the analysis of T-cell memory and the ways that T-cells control viruses that can cause tumors.

Presentation of the Nobel Prize will be made in December in Stockholm.

THE NOBEL PRIZE FOR MEDICINE

A Summary Of Dr. Peter Doherty's Honored Work

Dr. Peter Doherty, chairman of the immunology department at St. Jude Children's Research Hospital, has won the Nobel Prize for Medicine for his research that radically advanced the field of cellular immunology. He shares the prize with longtime collaborator Dr. Rolf Zinkernagel, director of the University of Zurich's Institute of Experimental Immunology. They performed pivotal experiments that first brought to light the fundamental requirements for T-cell initiation of an immune response. They showed T-cells must simultaneously recognize a foreign antigen and a self-protein of the Major Histocompatibility Complex on the surface of antigen-presenting cells.

The discovery by Drs. Doherty and Zinkernagel that MHC proteins restrict T-cell recognition of foreign antigens inaugurated a new era in immunology, an era of research that would clarify the functions of MHC proteins and their relationship to T cells. Innumerable insights into autoimmune diseases, graft rejection, organ transplantation and vaccine design emanate from the explanation of the role MHC proteins play in cell-mediated immunity.

Dr. Doherty's laboratories have continued to analyze the nature of virus-specific T-cell responses, collaborating extensively with Drs. Robert Webster and Alan Portner of St. Jude Hospital's virology/molecular biology department, Dr. John Sixbey of the hospital's infectious diseases department, Dr. James Ihle, chairman of the hospital's biochemistry department, and Dr. Gerald Grosveld, chairman of St. Jude's genetics department.

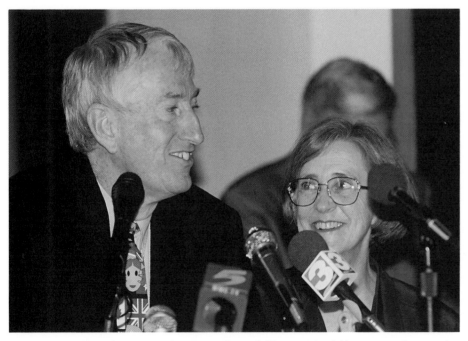

Dr. Doherty and his wife, Penny, at the news conference held at St. Jude Children's Research Hospital following the announcement that he had won the Nobel Prize for Medicine for 1996.